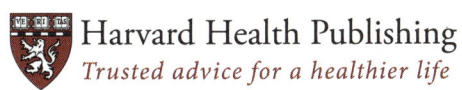

Dear Reader,

Core exercise has received a lot of publicity in recent years—much of it focusing on helping you flatten your belly or get washboard abs to show off on the beach. But there are many more reasons to pay attention to your core. Want to improve your running, swimming, golf, or tennis performance? Want to improve your posture, so you look younger and feel better? Want to build up your balance and stability so that you're less likely to fall? Want to make everyday acts like bending, turning, and reaching easier so that housework, fix-it projects, and gardening stay on your agenda? A strong, flexible core can help with all these goals—and it's the secret to sidestepping a lot of debilitating back pain. In short, core work is for everyone, no matter what age or fitness level.

Core muscles go far beyond the readily recognized "six-pack" abs that swimsuit models sport. Your core includes back, side, pelvic, and buttock muscles as well. It forms a sturdy central link between your upper and lower body. Much like the trunk of a young tree, core muscles need to be strong, yet flexible. A weak or inflexible core drains power from many of the movements you make.

Many people start core work by doing sit-ups or crunches. However, these are not the most effective moves for strengthening and toning your core. They target only one small part of the core—and instead of protecting your back, sit-ups may actually contribute to back or neck injuries. For this reason, this report focuses instead on core workouts that exercise all of your core muscles. What's more, you can do them on your own with little or no equipment, simply by following the instructions and photos in this report.

Our six core workouts feature exercises that facilitate moves you make during everyday life and sports. We've skipped standard crunches in favor of more effective exercises designed to strengthen more than one muscle group at a time. All of the exercises can be made easier or harder, depending on your current level of core fitness. We'll show you how to set achievable goals. Twenty to 40 minutes a few times a week—or even just five minutes a day—is all the time you need.

So flip through the pages of this report. Learn how core work can help you enjoy sports and daily activities, engage in the tasks you need to do with greater ease, and retain independence.

Sincerely,

Lauren E. Elson, M.D.
Medical Editor

Michele Stanten
Fitness Consultant

The importance of your core

Many people equate the core with their abdominal muscles. But your core is much more than that. It also includes muscles in your back, sides, pelvis, hips, and buttocks. These muscles are essential for movement and affect your everyday life in dozens of ways, large and small. This chapter will explain why it's worth the time to develop your core—and show you just what the core really is.

Why strengthen your core?

Think of your core muscles as the sturdy central link connecting your upper and lower body. Forces that propel movement either originate in your core or else transfer through it on the way from one part of the body to another. Weak, tight, or unbalanced core muscles can undermine the ease and power of the motions that are part of your everyday life.

When you toss a ball to a dog, for example, the complete arc of the movement (also known as the kinetic chain) should ideally run from the ground through your legs, hips, trunk and back, shoulder, elbow, and wrist in an even transfer of force. If there is a kink in the chain—such as weak core muscles—it undercuts the strength of the movement and may start a chain of misalignments in joints and limbs that can set you up for injuries over time.

No matter where a motion starts, it ripples upward and downward to adjoining links of the chain. Thus, weak or inflexible core muscles can impair how well your arms and legs function—and can sap power from many of the moves you make. In contrast, properly building up your core cranks up the power and enables you to go longer before fatigue sets in.

A strong core also enhances balance and stability. Therefore, it can help prevent falls and injuries during sports or other activities. In fact, a strong, flexible core underpins a healthy physique and, consequently, almost everything you do.

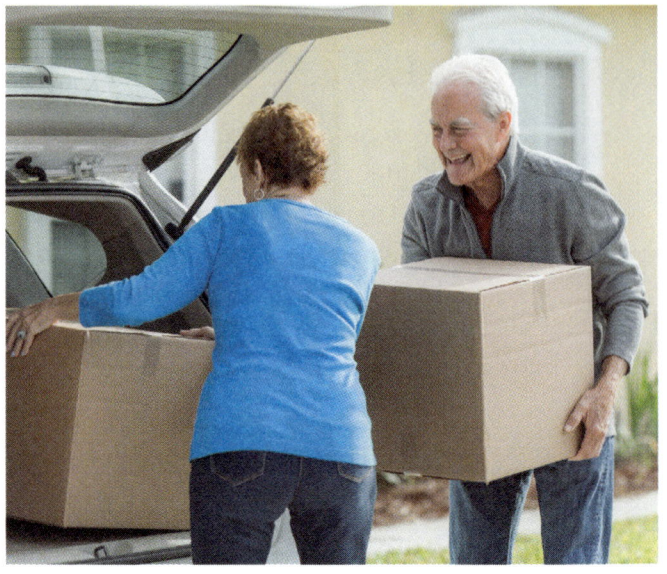

Core strength underlies just about everything you do, from jobs that involve lifting, twisting, and standing to sports like golf, tennis, and running. Even walking is easier when you engage your core muscles.

Everyday acts. Bending to scoop up a package, turning to look behind you, or simply standing in a line at the store—these are just a few of the many mundane actions that rely on your core and that you might not think about until they become difficult or painful. Basic activities of daily living—bathing or dressing, for example—call on your core.

On-the-job tasks. Jobs that involve lifting, twisting, and standing all depend on core muscles. But less strenuous tasks—like ones that involve sitting at your desk for hours—engage your core as well. Phone calls, typing, computer use, and similar work can make your back muscles surprisingly stiff and sore, particularly if you're not strong enough to practice good posture.

Sports and other pleasurable activities. Golf, tennis, badminton, biking, running, playing Frisbee, swimming, and many other athletic and recreational activities are powered by a strong core. Even getting up and down from the floor when playing with your kids or grandkids engages your core muscles. Less often mentioned are sexual activities, which call for core power and flexibility as well.

Housework, fix-it work, and gardening. Bending, lifting, twisting, carrying, hammering, reaching overhead—even vacuuming, mopping, and dusting are acts that spring from, or pass through, the core.

Core work also helps give you the following:

A healthy back. Low back pain—a debilitating, sometimes excruciating problem affecting four out of five Americans at some point in their lives—may be prevented by exercises that promote well-balanced, resilient core muscles. Moreover, when back pain strikes, a regimen of core exercises is often prescribed to relieve it, coupled with medications, physical therapy, or other treatments if necessary.

Balance and stability. Your core stabilizes your body, allowing you to move in any direction, even on the bumpiest terrain, or stand in one spot without losing your balance. As a result, core exercises can reduce your risk of falling.

Good posture. Weak core muscles contribute to slouching. Good posture trims your silhouette and projects confidence. More importantly, it lessens wear and tear on the spine, allows you to breathe deeply, and prevents the progression of spinal problems such as kyphosis (hunching of the back) and scoliosis (curvature of the spine). In one study, women with osteoporosis or osteopenia (the precursor to osteoporosis) gained almost a tenth of an inch in height after doing resistance exercises twice a week for eight months, while those who didn't exercise shrank an equivalent amount.

Stronger bones. Your spine, pelvis, and hip bones are some of the most common sites for osteoporosis-related fractures. The exercises that build core muscles tug on those bones, which signals your body to rein-

Figure 1: Front and back core muscles

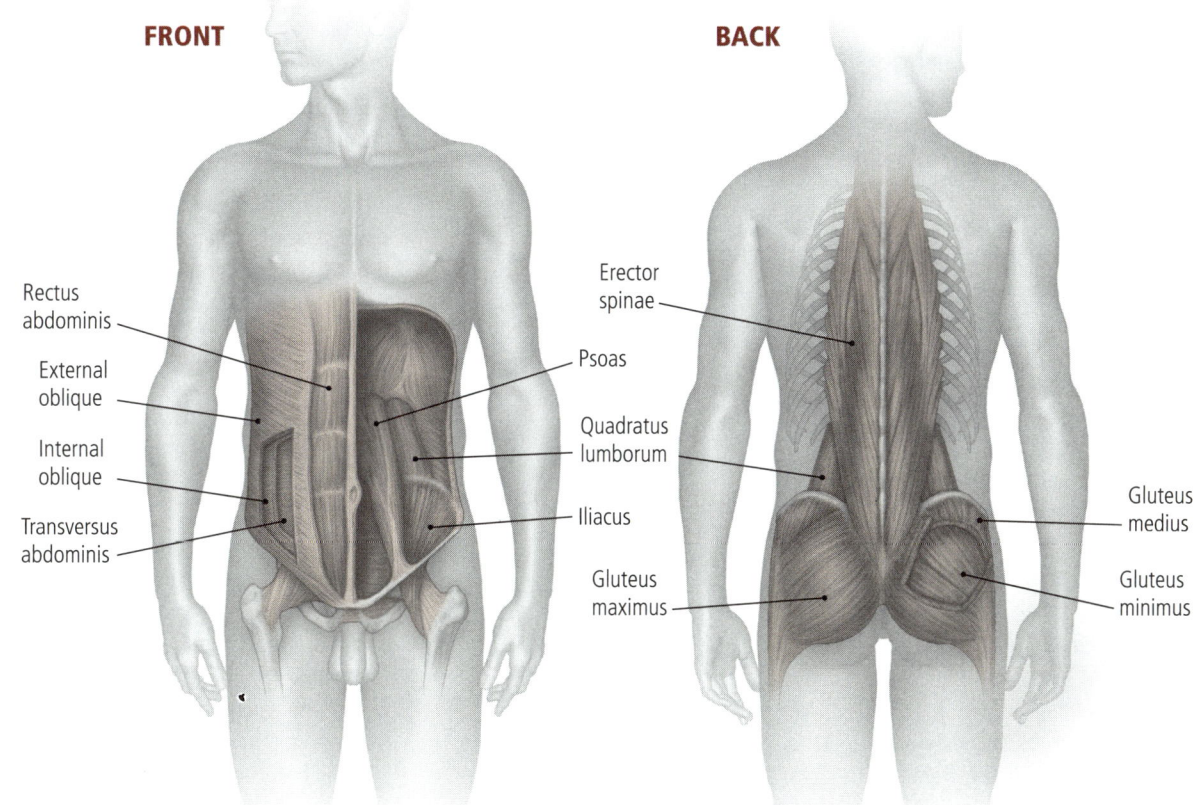

Your core is composed of many different muscles in the abdomen, back, sides, pelvis, hips, and buttocks. These muscles work together to support the spine and allow you to bend, twist, rotate, and stand upright.

force the bones, or at least slow the rate of bone loss that accompanies aging.

Major core muscles

Bounded largely by the rib cage and hips, your core spans muscles in your abdomen, back, sides, pelvis, buttocks, and hips (see Figure 1, page 3). In addition, a few muscles higher up on the back—the trapezius and latissimus dorsi—are supporting players that also contribute to core stability. Here is an introduction to the major muscles that our core workouts focus on.

In the abdomen

Exercise enthusiasts often use the word "abs" to refer to the rectus abdominis muscles, which create the "six-pack" sported by lean, chiseled athletes. But the abs are actually a quartet of abdominal muscle groups, all of which are important:

- Rectus abdominis (front)—a pair of long, vertical straps of muscle running from the sternum (breastbone) and ribs to the pubic bone. These muscles enable you to flex your trunk—for example, when you're getting out of bed in the morning.
- External obliques (both sides)—two large, flat muscles that enable you to twist your torso, as you do when reaching for something behind you or buckling your seat belt.
- Internal obliques (both sides, underneath the external obliques)—two smaller, flat muscles that work

---

Don't ignore your pelvic floor: Exercises to prevent or treat stress incontinence

One essential set of core muscles is often ignored even by exercise mavens. This sling of muscles and ligaments stretches from the pubic bone to the tailbone to form the pelvic floor. It helps support the bladder and other pelvic organs.

When you urinate, your body consciously relaxes the pelvic floor muscles and the two sphincter muscles that cinch the neck of the bladder. If pregnancy, childbirth, aging, or excess weight weakens the pelvic floor muscles, one set of roadblocks that helps prevent urine leaks is compromised, and the bladder may slip downward. Often, leaks start occurring when you jump, cough, laugh, or exert yourself in ways that put pressure on your abdomen. This common problem is called stress incontinence.

Strengthening the pelvic floor muscles can help relieve stress incontinence in many women. A trial from the Netherlands found that it can also help reduce symptoms of pelvic organ prolapse in women. In men, strengthening these muscles helps cut urine leaks after prostate surgery, especially when combined with other behavioral strategies, such as avoiding caffeine and alcohol. Other research has found that strengthening these muscles could also help alleviate lower back pain.

Whether or not you experience incontinence, pelvic floor exercises can help improve sexual fitness by enhancing the rigidity of the penis during intercourse and also tightening the vagina.

Find the right muscles

Kegel exercises can help tune up pelvic floor muscles if done regularly. First, you need to pinpoint the right muscles by following these directions.

Make sure you're starting with an empty bladder. Tighten up the muscles you would use to avoid passing gas. If you're a woman, it may help to imagine tightening your vagina around a tampon. (An older tip—engaging the muscles you use to stop a stream of urine—has been discredited.) Generally, you should feel like you are pulling in the anal area.

Now practice tightening up, holding, and releasing the muscles. As you do this, try not to contract abdominal or leg muscles—or, indeed, any other muscles. It may help to put your hand on your belly so you can sense whether you're tightening your abs. If you're still not sure you have the right set of muscles, biofeedback can help you learn to do Kegels correctly. Talk to your doctor about this.

How to do pelvic floor exercises

Pull in the pelvic floor muscles as described above. Hold for a count of three to five. Release and relax for a count of three to five. Do 10 to 15 times. Practice these exercises three times a day, preferably once while lying down, once while sitting, and once while standing.

While pelvic floor exercises may take three to six weeks to work, you may notice improvement earlier.

Need more help?

Talk to your doctor about other options if these exercises aren't enough. Reasons for urinary incontinence vary, and more than one problem may be involved. A thorough exam will help determine causes and identify the right treatment. Often, a doctor can suggest healthy habits and behavioral changes to help curb urine leaks, possibly in combination with medications, surgery, or other strategies.

in tandem with the external obliques to enable you to twist your torso. (The main difference is that the external obliques handle rotation on the opposite side, while internal obliques handle rotation on the same side—so that twisting to the left to pass food at the table or run the vacuum cleaner, for example, would involve the right external and left internal obliques.)

- Transversus abdominis (front and sides, underneath the internal obliques)—a wide, flat girdle of muscle wrapping around the torso that is a key spinal stabilizer. It holds in the internal organs when

Your waistline: A measure of health

If you're like many people, your most obvious core concern may be your waistline. It's not just a cosmetic issue. The Nurses' Health Study, a major long-term trial, showed that participants with larger waists had a greater risk of dying from heart disease or cancer, or dying prematurely from any cause. The larger the waist, the higher the risk. Even those at a healthy weight had a higher risk of dying from heart disease if their weight was distributed so that it concentrated in a muffin top.

You may wonder why belly fat is so worrisome. It has to do with the nature of the fat. There are two types of belly fat. Subcutaneous fat lies near the surface, tucked between abdominal skin and a wall of muscle. While it may not look so good, subcutaneous fat is relatively benign. But the other type of belly fat, called visceral fat, lies beneath those muscles, surrounding vital abdominal organs. Biologically, visceral fat is far more dangerous than subcutaneous fat because visceral fat isn't just a storage depot for calories. It actually produces compounds that contribute to insulin resistance, lipid imbalances (like too much harmful LDL cholesterol and too little helpful HDL cholesterol), and inflammation, all of which fuel heart disease, diabetes, and certain cancers.

How big a waist measurement is unhealthy? A panel at the National Institutes of Health set the danger mark at 35 inches for women and 40 inches for men. But some public health officials think the guidelines should be stricter than that. An international study of more than 168,000 people in 63 countries pegged entry to the danger zone at 31.5 inches in women and 37 inches in men.

What helps?

You can't spot-reduce your way to a smaller waist. Getting sufficient aerobic exercise, however, can help shave fat off your entire body, including worrisome visceral fat. A four-pronged approach will set you up for success:

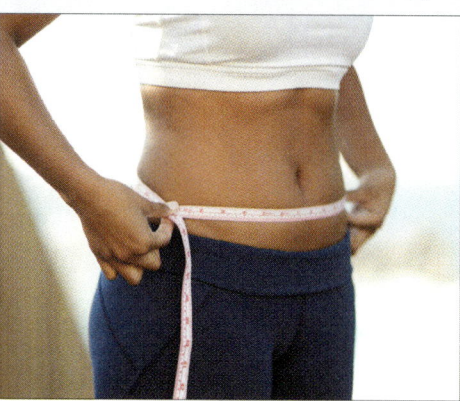

How to measure your waist correctly
- Put a tape measure around your waist just above your hip bones.
- Make sure the tape measure is parallel to the floor and snug, but not compressing the skin.
- Breathe out and measure.

Eating habits. If you need to lose weight, eat mindfully and burn more calories than you take in. Emphasize vitamin-packed vegetables and fruits; whole grains; fish, lean poultry, and beans and other legumes as lean protein sources; plus healthy fats found in many nuts and in olive, canola, soy, sunflower, and peanut oils. Cut back on unnecessary calories from sweets, sodas, refined grains like white bread or white rice, saturated fats and trans fats, fried and fast foods, and mindless snacking. And keep a close eye on portion sizes.

Aerobic exercise. Regularly engage in moderate to vigorous aerobic exercise (walking, jogging, swimming, biking, rowing), which works many muscles, including those of the core, while burning calories at a faster clip than isolated core work. This helps decrease total body fat and abdominal fat even in the absence of weight loss. Aim for two-and-a-half to five hours every week of moderate activity (such as brisk walking at 3 to 4 mph), or vigorous exercise (jogging at 5 to 6 mph) for half that time.

Sleep. Getting the right amount each night—not too much and not too little—will make it easier to keep your waistline trim. People who averaged six or fewer hours of sleep a night gained 66% more visceral fat than those who snoozed seven to eight hours, according to a study published in the journal *Obesity*. At the opposite end of the spectrum, a separate study of 293 adults found that people averaging nine or more hours a night gained 43% more visceral fat. Aim to get seven to eight hours of shut-eye a night if you want to maintain or shrink your waistline.

Stress reduction. When you're stressed out, your body releases the hormone cortisol, which is associated with abdominal fat. In studies, people with chronic stress or those who've experienced stressful events have been found to have larger waistlines and more visceral fat. Activities like yoga, deep breathing, and meditation have been shown in studies to reduce stress and lower cortisol.

you're sitting or standing, so it's working even when you're not moving.

In the back
The erector spinae, a group of vertical muscles collectively stretching along the entire spine, help you straighten up and stand upright with good posture.

In the pelvis, buttocks, and hips
The muscles in this region straddle the realm from the hips to the back and also include the three sets of muscles in the buttocks that are known informally as the "gluteals" or "glutes."

- Gluteus maximus (buttocks)—two bulky muscles that permit you to powerfully extend the hip and rotate the thigh, providing power for walking and climbing stairs.
- Gluteus medius and minimus (buttocks)—four fan-shaped muscles that let you rotate the hip, push the thigh away from the centerline of your body, and stabilize your pelvis while standing, especially when balancing on one leg. Strengthening these muscles can also prevent or help with knee and back issues.
- Iliopsoas (pelvis and hips)—this muscle group is made up of two muscles, the iliacus and the psoas, that reach down from the mid-spine and wrap around the hip joint to the thighbone, allowing you to lift your legs and remain stable while standing. These muscles help you pick up your legs when you go up steps.
- Quadratus lumborum (pelvis and back)—either of two straps of muscle (one on each side of the body) that stabilize the pelvis and lower spine and permit you to bend to the sides and slightly backward, as well as hike up each hip. They stabilize you while doing activities like housecleaning.

Beyond muscles
Though the core is essential for all full-body movements, your core muscles can't do all the work by themselves. The spine, pelvis, and hip joints, plus other structures in your body's core, are equally important for standing, sitting, and moving.

Thirty-three interlocked vertebrae form the spine, a bony column that flexes along nearly all of its length. Vertebrae are divided into five regions. The top three regions are the cervical spine (neck), the thoracic spine (upper and mid-back), and the lumbar spine, the hot spot for lower back injuries and pain (see Figure 2, at left). Sandwiched between the vertebrae in these regions are shock-absorbing discs that enable mobility. The bottom two regions form the sacrum, a triangular bone that connects to the pelvic girdle, and the short tail of the coccyx. Both consist of fused vertebrae and

Figure 2: Regions of the spine

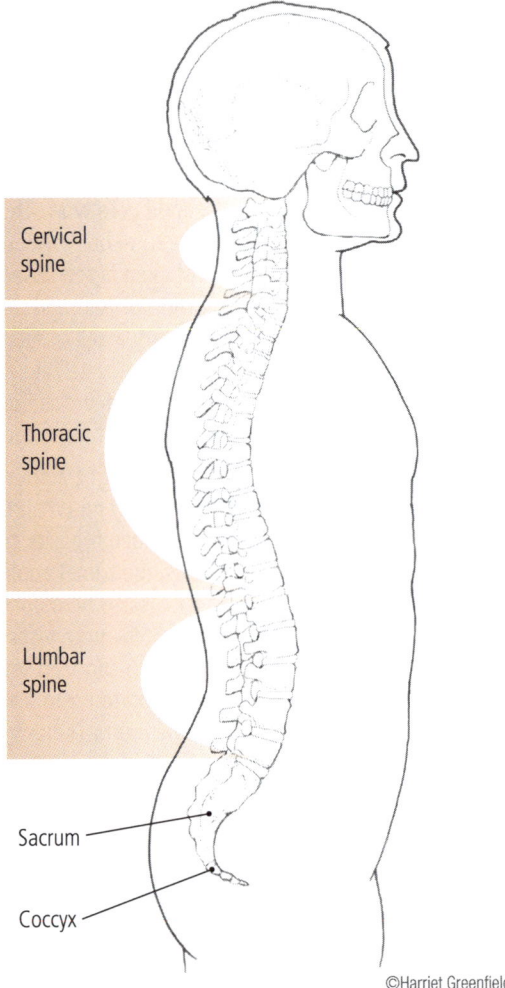

Core work supports the spine, especially the thoracic and lumbar regions. Low back pain often originates in the lumbar area, which extends from the bottom of your rib cage to your sacrum (the triangular bone found between your hip bones) and includes the lowest five mobile vertebrae.

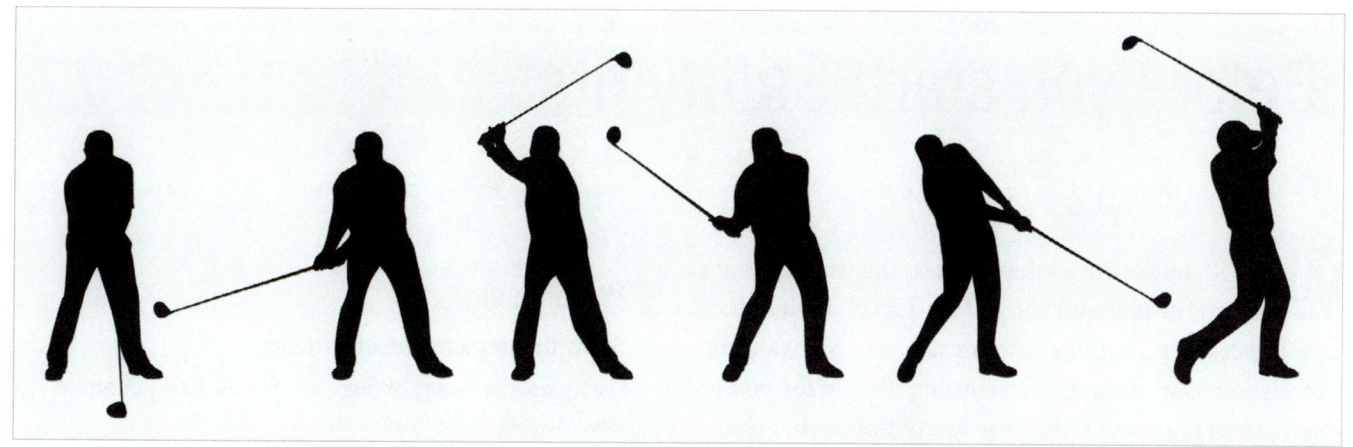

When you swing at a golf ball, the complete arc of the movement (the kinetic chain) should ideally run from the ground through your legs, hips, trunk and back, shoulders, and arms in an even transfer of force. Weak core muscles undercut the strength of the movement.

no discs, so this part of the spine is not flexible.

The bony girdle of the pelvis acts as the base of your core. The hip joints—two sockets that the balls at the top of the thighbones fit into neatly—are situated in the lower third of the pelvis, toward the front.

Inside each hip joint, tough, flexible tissue called cartilage cushions the junctions between bones and absorbs synovial fluid, a lubricant that helps protect against the wear and tear of friction. Ligaments made of strong, usually inelastic, tissue bind and stabilize the joint.

Throughout your core, stretchy cords of tissue called tendons tether muscle to bone and cartilage. Your brain coordinates lightning-quick signals passing along nerve pathways that instruct muscles to contract and relax. The muscles tug on tendons attached to bones, allowing you to move in a multitude of ways—to walk and jump, dance and run, twist and bend.

Before you start: Safety first

While it's tempting to skip right to the workouts, it's best to think about safety first. Check with a doctor, if necessary, to make sure it's safe for you to do the exercises in our workouts. Assuming it's safe for you to begin, then read and follow the safety tips in this chapter and in "Posture, alignment, and angles," page 11. Core work is subtle, so look carefully at our pointers on good form in the exercise instructions. Finally, it's important to be aware of the warning signs (at right) that should prompt a call to 911 if you experience any of these while exercising or shortly afterward.

When to check with a doctor first

Should you check with a doctor before launching into a core workout? Generally, light to moderate exercise is safe for healthy adults. If you engage in regular activity, odds are good you can undertake the workouts without difficulty. But it's best to talk to a doctor first if any of the following apply:

- You've had hip surgery.
- You've got pain in your hip joints or back.
- You have a chronic or unstable health condition, such as heart disease or several risk factors for heart disease, a respiratory ailment, high blood pressure, osteoporosis, or diabetes.

The Get Active Questionnaire, a tool developed by the Canadian Society for Exercise Physiology, can help you determine whether you should talk to your doctor before embarking on, or ramping up, any exercise program. You can find it at www.health.harvard.edu/GAQ.

If you do need to speak to a doctor, show him or her the core workout pages in this report and ask if you can safely follow the program that's laid out here. Your doctor may feel that the exercises are fine, or may modify a workout to make it safer for you. If you need a less intense core workout, you may want to refer to *Gentle Core Exercises*, another Harvard Medical School Special Health Report. (See the

▶ Warning signs

Signs that indicate an emergency

If you experience any of these symptoms during or after exercise, call 911 immediately:

- chest pain, pressure, heaviness, or tightness
- faintness or loss of consciousness
- significant or persistent shortness of breath or dizziness.

Ask your doctor whether any other warning signs specific to your health history warrant a call.

Signs that should prompt a call to your doctor

Persistent or intense muscle pain that starts during a session or right afterward, or muscle soreness that persists more than one to two weeks, merits a call to your doctor for advice. (This is in contrast to the normal muscle soreness that starts 12 to 48 hours after an exercise session and gradually abates.) You should also call your doctor if a routine you've been doing for a while without discomfort starts to cause you pain.

"Resources" section, page 52, for more information.)

If necessary, your doctor can refer you to a physical therapist, a physiatrist (a physician who specializes in physical medicine and rehabilitation), or another specialist for further evaluation. These professionals can help you tailor an exercise program to your needs if you're recovering from surgery or injuries, or if you have chronic problems that interfere with exercise by sparking pain or limiting movements. They can also tell you whether certain types of exercises will be helpful or harmful given your situation. Usually, you'll be able to find safe, enjoyable activities, though some precautions may be in order.

Occasionally, a doctor may recommend working out with the supervision of an experienced personal trainer to help ensure that you're doing exercises properly. While encouraging and motivating you, trainers can fine-tune your form, especially helpful in core work because subtle movements can make an

The right (and wrong) way to do three classic core moves

Good form is crucial to protecting yourself from injury and getting the most benefit from an exercise. Here's a look at the right and wrong way to perform three exercises that are fundamental to a good core workout.

PLANK
Tips and techniques:
- *Do* form a straight line from head to heels.
- *Don't* bend at your hips.
- *Don't* let your belly drop toward the floor.

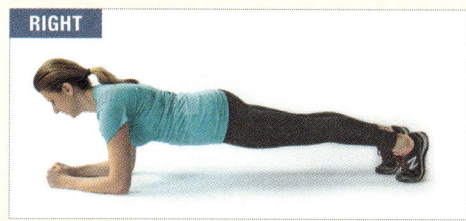

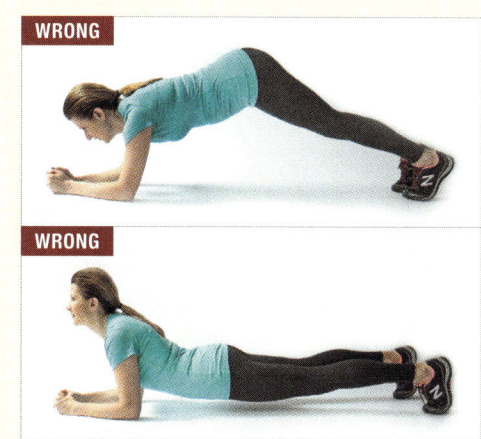

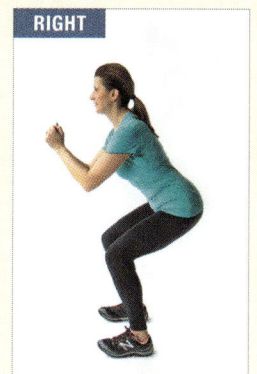

SQUAT
Tips and techniques:
- *Do* bend at your hips.
- *Do* lean forward about 45°.
- *Don't* let your knees go farther forward than your toes.
- *Don't* round your back.

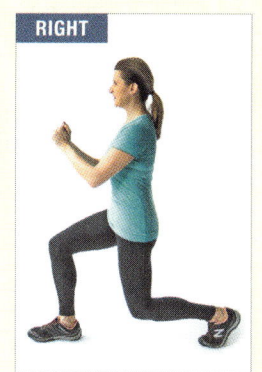
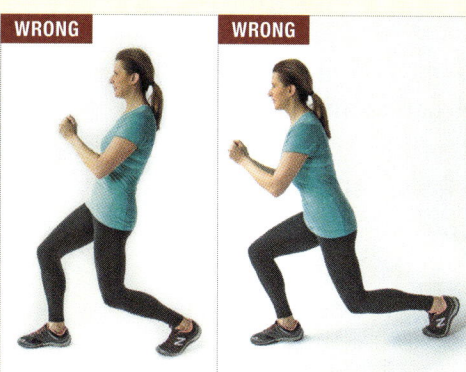

LUNGE
Tips and techniques:
- *Do* keep your front knee over your ankle.
- *Don't* lean back.
- *Don't* lean forward.

---

exercise effective or ineffective. Personal trainers teach new skills, change up routines to beat boredom, and safely push you to the next level. No national licensing requirements exist for personal trainers, although standards for the accrediting fitness organizations that train them have been set by the National Commission for Certifying Agencies. Two well-respected organizations that offer certification and programs of study for personal trainers are the American College of Sports Medicine (ACSM) and the American Council on Exercise (ACE); others include the National Council on Strength and Fitness (NCSF), the National Strength and Conditioning Association (NSCA), and the National Academy of Sports Medicine (NASM).

All fitness organizations have different requirements for training and expertise. Some trainers specialize in working with particular populations—for example, athletes or older adults—and may have taken courses and possibly certifying exams in those areas.

12 tips for exercising safely and effectively

1. Warm up. Before a full core workout, march in place for several minutes while swinging your arms, or dance to a few songs. It's safe to skip this if you've already warmed up through other activities.

2. Form first. Good form means aligning your body as

described in the exercise instructions and moving smoothly through an exercise. Read the "Tips and techniques" section of each exercise for advice on correct alignment. Also see "The right (and wrong) way to do three classic core moves," page 9.

3. **Reps second.** Quality trumps quantity. Do only as many reps as you can manage with excellent form (see "Posture, alignment, and angles," page 11). And don't hold a position longer than you're able to do it with proper form. Work up to the full number of reps or seconds gradually. Once you can do a full set, consider adding another (up to three sets).

4. **Feel no pain.** Core work shouldn't hurt. Stop if you feel sharp or intense pain, especially in the lower back. Check your form and try again. If the pain persists, check with a doctor or therapist before repeating the move. (Later discomfort from muscle fatigue is normal; see "Feeling sore?" at right.)

5. **Practice often.** You'll see the best gains if you consistently do core exercises three times a week.

6. **Photos tell only part of the story.** Photos can make core work look easier than it actually is. Carefully read the instructions and the "Tips and techniques" section of each exercise.

7. **Brace yourself.** Tighten your core muscles before starting the movement described in each exercise. Here's how: while sitting, standing, or lying on your back, gently but firmly tighten your abdominal muscles. Once you're braced, a gentle push from any direction should not cause you to lose your balance. Some trainers suggest imagining that you're pulling in your muscles to zip up a tight pair of jeans and fasten a tight jacket. Try bracing or zipping up for 10 seconds at a time while breathing normally.

8. **Reach beyond abs.** Having a rippling six-pack but a weak back is a recipe for disaster. So don't just focus on abdominal exercises that create a buff appearance. The program in this report works all your core muscles—protecting your back, powering everyday activities, and boosting sports performance.

9. **Be flexible.** Core flexibility is as important as core strength. In fact, too much strength without flexibility can make your back throb and interfere with smooth, powerful moves in sports like tennis and golf. So don't skimp on stretches. You'll find a section on stretches in this report at the end of the workouts (see "Finish with stretches," page 43).

10. **Start with stability, then add instability.** Master exercise movement patterns, such as lunges, bridges, and planks, on a flat, stable surface. Core work gets harder when an unstable surface, such as a stability ball or Bosu, is introduced, because your muscles have to work harder to hold a position steadily or stabilize you while moving. Take time to perfect difficult exercises on a stable surface before shifting to an unstable one.

11. **If it's too hard, drop down.** Do fewer reps or hold for fewer seconds. Still too difficult? Try the easier variation in the "Make it easier" section for each exercise. If you're still struggling, try fewer reps (or seconds) of the easier variation.

12. **If it's too easy, move up.** As it becomes easier to do exercises with excellent form, begin adding reps (up to 10) or seconds. Next, add sets or try the harder variation in the "Make it harder" section for each exercise. As you move up to more challenging exercises, leave the simpler ones behind.

Feeling sore?

When you crank up physical activity by doing a new set of exercises, your muscles are likely to feel sore the next day or two. Delayed-onset muscle soreness is a normal response to taxing muscles. Usually, it peaks 24 to 48 hours after a workout before gradually easing, then disappears entirely in another day or so. By contrast, sudden, sharp, or long-lasting pain should prompt you to call a doctor for advice (see "Warning signs," page 8).

If your muscles feel really sore a day or two after a core workout, you probably overdid it. Dial down your core work next time. Try to finish just one full set of each exercise in the workout. Still too much for your muscles? Do fewer reps of the exercises you find especially hard. Then build up gradually.

For example, instead of trying to do four front planks a day, start with one. Try this for a few days, then add a second plank. When you're comfortable at that level—that is, not feeling a lot of muscle soreness—add a third plank. And so on. If even one plank knocks you out, dial down the number of seconds you hold it: instead of 30 seconds, try 10 seconds for several days, then try 15 or 20 seconds. And so on.

Posture, alignment, and angles: Striking the right pose

Posture counts for a lot when you're exercising. Aligning your body properly is the key to good form, which nets you greater gains and fewer injuries. In fact, good posture helps any time you're moving. If one foot is always turned slightly inward, for example, it impedes power whether you're walking, climbing the stairs, jogging, or playing sports. Worse, it paves the way for injuries to the ankle, knee, hip, and beyond, since the effects of this physical quirk can zigzag their way up your body. Similarly, sitting up straight and comfortably aligned in a chair can make desk work feel less tiresome. Hours of computer and desk work tend to make your shoulders hunch and your head and neck jut forward uncomfortably.

Committing to core work will do much to improve your posture whether you're sitting, standing, or moving. A well-rounded set of exercises that targets all the core muscles is best. If you only work on strengthening abs, your back muscles will grow weaker by comparison. Then, instead of standing straight, your body will curve forward. Likewise, posture is thrown out of kilter when muscles lose flexibility, becoming tighter and eventually shortening so that your range of motion is increasingly limited. Among other problems, this can cause back pain.

Our workouts are designed to build strength and flexibility in all your major core muscles. Doing any of our full workouts, or the moves in our four short workouts, can help you avoid such problems.

Posture checks

Quick posture checks before and during exercise can help you avoid injury and squeeze the most benefit from your workout. If possible (mainly when doing standing exercises), look in a mirror from time to time. Try to take a few moments each day to practice better posture, too. When exercise instructions in our workouts ask you to stand up straight, that means the following:

- chin parallel to the floor
- shoulders back and down
- arms at your sides, elbows relaxed
- abdominal muscles pulled in
- knees pointing straight ahead
- feet pointing straight ahead
- body weight evenly distributed on both feet.

Stay neutral

Whether you're standing or seated, neutral posture requires you to keep your chin parallel to the floor; your shoulders, hips, and knees at even heights; and your knees and feet pointing straight ahead.

A neutral spine takes into account the slight natural curves of the spine—it's not flexed or arched to overemphasize the curve of the lower back. One way to find neutral is to tip your pelvis forward as far as is comfortable (lifting your tailbone up), then tip it backward (tucking your tailbone under) as far as is comfortable. The spot approximately in the middle is neutral. If you're not used to standing or sitting up straight, it may take a while for this to feel natural.

A neutral wrist is firm and straight, not bent.

Neutral alignment means keeping your body in a straight line from head to toe except for the slight natural curves of the spine.

Get the angle

When angles appear in exercise instructions, use these tips. Try visualizing a 90° angle as an L or two adjacent sides of a square, or picture the distance between the minute hand and hour hand of a clock at 3 o'clock. To visualize a 45° angle, mentally slice the 90° angle in half. ▼

Getting started

Where should core work fit into your exercise plans? What equipment, if any, will you need? This chapter answers those questions and explains the basic terminology used in the six core workouts.

To set goals and keep track of your progress, see the Special Section, "Setting goals, motivating yourself, and maintaining gains," starting on page 46.

Which workout should you do?

Start with the Standing Core Workout (page 18), the Floor Core Workout (page 22), or the Pilates Workout (page 26), in which you'll learn key exercises on a flat, stable surface. Once you master those three routines, you can move on to the Medicine Ball, Stability Ball, and Bosu workouts. Holding a medicine ball for resistance or introducing an unstable surface, such as a stability ball or Bosu, turns the challenge up several notches because your muscles have to work harder. Changing workouts occasionally can also help keep you motivated. Just don't attempt those workouts until you've perfected the simpler ones.

How does core work fit into your exercise plans?

You should aim to do a full core workout two or three times a week. But fitting core work into a broader exercise program will give you the biggest bang for your buck in terms of health benefits (see "Beyond the core: Why exercise?" below). A well-rounded exercise plan has several facets, according to the Physical Activity Guidelines for Americans, issued by the U.S. Department of Health and Human Services. The

---

Beyond the core: Why exercise?

Whether you find the government's Physical Activity Guidelines for Americans exhilarating or exhausting, following that prescription for regular exercise will help you feel, think, and look better. Exercise can take a load off aching joints by strengthening muscles and chipping away at excess pounds. Or it can help you avoid gaining weight or prevent pounds you've lost from sneaking back on again. Regular exercise enables some people to cut back on medications they take, such as drugs for high blood pressure or diabetes. And that can ease unwelcome side effects and save money.

Strong evidence from thousands of studies shows that engaging in regular exercise offers a host of health benefits beyond those already discussed for core workouts.

Regular exercise
- lowers your risks for early death, heart disease, stroke, type 2 diabetes, high blood pressure, high cholesterol, and metabolic syndrome (a complex problem that increases the risk for stroke, heart disease, and diabetes by blending three or more of the following factors: high blood pressure, high triglycerides, low HDL cholesterol, a large waistline, and difficulty regulating blood sugar)
- reduces your risk of developing certain types of cancer, including colorectal, breast, bladder, endometrial, esophageal, kidney, lung, and stomach
- strengthens muscles, lungs, and heart
- helps prevent falls that can lead to debilitating fractures and loss of independence
- helps prevent weight gain
- may aid weight loss when combined with the proper diet
- promotes better sleep
- eases depression, stress, and anxiety
- boosts mental sharpness in older adults and reduces the risk of dementia
- improves functional abilities in older adults—that is, being able to walk up stairs, heft groceries, rise from a chair without help, and perform a multitude of other activities that permit independence or bring joy to life
- helps maintain strong bones (provided the exercises are weight-bearing, meaning they work against gravity)
- lowers the risk for hip fractures.

guidelines include the following recommendations:
- Accumulate at least two-and-a-half hours (150 minutes) of moderate aerobic activity per week, or one-and-a-quarter hours (75 minutes) of vigorous activity per week. During moderate activity you can talk, but not sing; during vigorous activity you can't say more than a few words without catching your breath. Walking, running, biking, swimming, cross-country skiing, tennis, rowing, and many additional activities offer aerobic benefits.
- Do strength-training sessions two or three times a week for all major muscle groups, including your core.
- If you're an older adult at risk for falling, add balance exercises.

Core work falls under the second and third categories: strength training and enhancing balance. Many of the exercises we've selected tone more than just core muscles: for example, lunges strengthen your legs, while planks work some arm and back muscles. But to target all the major muscle groups, you need to do some additional exercises, too. For example, supplement the Floor Core Workout with squats or lunges to strengthen your lower body. Add push-ups, rows, biceps curls, and triceps extensions to the other core routines to strengthen the upper body.

Within reason, the more challenging core work you do, the greater your gains will be. So, for example, you'll see better results—such as more power in your golf or tennis game or a more toned look to your muscles—if you're using our workouts two or three times a week or adding bursts of core exercise daily than if you include just a few extra core exercises in your twice-weekly strength-training sessions. Still, even a little core work, such as a few planks twice a week, is better than none.

If you're a serious athlete or have set your sights on competing in a marathon, 5K, or sprint triathlon, core work should be part of your routine. Sports medicine experts encourage athletes to rotate exercise routines involving different parts of the body. This builds power while putting less stress on joints and reducing overuse injuries. Consult with a personal trainer, who can help you build a safe, complete program aimed at achieving your goals.

Four short workouts

Try these on busy days, or when you just need a change.

The first two workouts use only body weight for resistance and are performed on a stable surface, which makes it easier to master the movements. The third includes moves that work your upper and lower body at the same time for better balance and coordination, while the fourth features advanced exercises. As always, repeat only as many times (or hold for as many seconds) as is possible with good form. Remember to warm up first for several minutes and stretch afterward.

1 Short workout

Bridge, page 22

Opposite arm and leg raise, page 24

Side squat with knee lift, page 20

2 Short workout

Side plank, page 25

Alternating reverse lunge, page 19

Alternating toe taps, page 23

3 Short combo workout

Cross chop and lift, page 31

Lunge with rotation, page 32

Bridge with pullover, page 34

4 Short challenge workout

Single-leg stance with medicine ball, page 34

Bridge extensions and curls, page 38

Reverse lunge with rotation, page 40

Finding the time

For full workouts, such as the Standing Core Workout, estimate 20 minutes for one set of exercises and stretches or 40 minutes for two sets. But even when you don't have time to do one of the full routines, you can sneak in some core exercises in as little as five to 10 minutes. Here are some suggestions.

Try a shorter workout. Our four short workouts (above) represent less of a time commitment than a full workout. Start with workout 1 or 2, since both are on a stable surface, before attempting the additional challenges of the medicine ball, Bosu, or stability ball in workouts 3 and 4. Or mix or match three or four exercises from any of the routines to create your own short workout.

Fit in bursts of exercise. Even the busiest people have moments of downtime during the day. Challenge yourself to see how often you can slip in a burst of core work. Can you do one or two moves before leaving home in the morning? How about during TV commercial breaks? Can you close your office door at work and do a few squats and lunges while talking on the phone? Start slowly by writing a reminder on your calendar—say, every Monday and Thursday—then gradually fold bursts of core exercise into additional days.

Choose cues to prompt activity. Identify predictable wait times or other recurring events that can serve as triggers for specific exercises. While waiting for the light to change, for example, check your posture or practice bracing yourself (see "Brace yourself," page 10). While your computer is firing up, try a few front planks, side squats with knee lifts, or pliés. When you finish a task, take an active break by doing side leg lifts or reverse lunges.

Incorporate core exercises into strength sessions. Add two to four core exercises to your twice-weekly strength-training sessions. This option is an excellent fallback position during especially busy weeks. When you're not as busy, try to step it up again by doing a full core workout.

The right stuff: Choosing equipment

You needn't spend a cent on fancy equipment to get a good workout. Our Standing Core Workout (page 18), Floor Core Workout (page 22), and Pilates Workout (page 26) rely on body weight alone. The other workouts in this report do require some equipment, however. Consider buying just enough for the workout you'd like to do next, and investing in the rest later, as you move on to other workouts. Or, if you have a gym membership, use the facility's equipment. In the following list, you'll find descriptions of the equipment used in the six workouts in this report. All of the products are available online or wherever fitness products are sold.

Chair. Choose a sturdy chair that won't tip over easily. A plain wooden dining chair without arms or heavy padding works well.

Mat. Choose a nonslip, well-padded mat. Prices start at about $20. A thick carpet will do in a pinch.

Yoga strap. This is a non-elastic cotton or nylon strap of six feet or longer that helps you position your body properly during certain stretches or while doing the easier variation of a stretch. A strap with a D-ring or buckle fastener on one end allows you to put a loop around a foot or leg and then grasp the other end of the strap. Prices start at about $7. A belt or bathrobe tie can also be used.

Medicine ball. Similar in size to a soccer ball or basketball, medicine balls come in different weights. Some have a handle on top. A 4-pound to 6-pound medicine ball is a good start for most people. Some bounce when you drop them and will roll. Non-bouncing ones will stay where they land. You can use either for the Medicine Ball Workout (page 31) in this report. Your choice of a ball will only affect how you execute the overhead slam exercise (page 33); you'll have to catch or chase a bouncing ball, while you'll have to squat down to pick up a non-bouncing one. Prices start at about $20.

Stability ball. Large, inflatable orbs called stability balls come in several sizes (55, 65, and 75 centi-

---

Why not just do a few sit-ups?

Once, sit-ups ruled in dusty school gyms, and planks were merely flooring. Now planks have claimed the spotlight as core workout stars while old standards like sit-ups and crunches have fallen out of favor. Why the shift?

First, sit-ups may hurt your back by pushing your curved spine against the floor, and also by overworking the hip flexor muscles, which run from the thighs to the lumbar spine (in the lower back). When these muscles are too strong or overly tight, they tug on lumbar vertebrae, which can be a source of lower back discomfort.

Second, planks recruit a better balance of muscles on the front, sides, and back of the body than sit-ups, which target just a few muscles.

Third, daily activities and athletics call on your muscles to work together, not in isolation. Sit-ups or crunches cherry-pick just a few muscle groups to strengthen. Our core workouts stress dynamic patterns of movement used in many activities that build up your entire core.

meters are most common, but smaller and larger balls are available). To select a ball, check the package for a size chart based on your height. When you sit on a ball, your hips and knees should be at 90° angles. Air pressure counts: a firmer ball makes an exercise more challenging; a softer ball makes an exercise easier to do. Prices start at about $20.

Bosu. A Bosu Balance Trainer is essentially half a stability ball mounted on a heavy rubber platform that helps hold it firmly in place. Fully inflate the Bosu to nine inches in height. It should be firm to the touch, but not overinflated. Prices start at about $120.

Terminology used in the workouts

As you'll see, our exercise instructions include specific terminology, which is explained below.

Repetitions (reps). Each rep is a single, complete exercise. If you cannot do all the reps at first, do as many as you can manage with good form. Gradually increase the number of reps as you improve.

Set. A specific number of repetitions make a set. In our core workouts, a set is usually 10 reps. Generally, we suggest doing one to three sets. Just as with reps, only do the number of sets you can manage with good form and work your way up over time.

Tempo. This provides a count for the key movements in an exercise. For example, a 3–3 tempo means that you count to three as you perform an exercise, such as lowering into a squat, then count to three as you return to the starting position. A 3–1–3 tempo means that you will also count while holding a position—for example, counting to three while extending one arm and one leg, holding for a count of one, then counting to three as you return to the starting position. To avoid hurrying, it helps to count while watching or listening to seconds tick by on a clock. When you can no longer maintain the recommended tempo, your muscles are fatigued. Stop that particular exercise, even if you haven't finished all of the reps.

Hold. Hold tells you the number of seconds to pause while holding a pose during an exercise. You'll see this in stretches, which are held for up to 30 sec-

> ### Building a better six-pack
>
> Given all the time and energy it takes, creating six-pack abs ought to be considered a sport in itself.
>
> First, you need to build up specific muscles—it's the ripples in the rectus abdominis, after all, that form that pleasing washboard silhouette. Among other key muscles are the obliques on each side; the transversus abdominis, which girdles the waist; the erector spinae, which support the spine; and the quadratus lumborum, which stabilizes the pelvis (see Figure 1, page 3).
>
> Second, you have to pare body fat to a minimum in order to show off even the buffest abs. And spot reducing isn't possible. To lose a layer of fat, you'll need to exercise restraint at the table, plus do sufficient aerobic work, such as walking, running, swimming, cycling, or Zumba. Interval training, which varies higher- and lower-intensity aerobic activities during a workout, can be especially helpful.
>
> Still interested? Talk to an experienced personal trainer, who can tailor a program of aerobic exercise, healthy eating, and challenging strength and core moves.

onds, and in plank exercises, for example. Start with a comfortable number of seconds, then work up. Holding for the full time recommended will give you the best results from the stretch or exercise.

Rest. Resting gives your muscles a chance to recharge, which helps you maintain good form. We specify a range of time to rest between sets, or sometimes between reps for especially tiring exercises like planks. How much of this time you need will differ depending on your level of fitness and the intensity of the exercises. No rest is needed during warm-ups and stretches.

Starting position. This describes how to position your body before starting the movement of the exercise.

Movement. This explains how to perform one complete repetition correctly.

Tips and techniques. We offer two or three pointers to help you maintain good form and reap the greatest gains from the exercise.

Make it easier. This gives you an option to modify the exercise when it is too difficult.

Make it harder. This gives you an option to modify the exercise when it is too easy.

Measuring gains

You don't need to wait very long to notice results from core work. If you do core exercises consistently, you will start to see progress in as little as two weeks. The more you step up your program by challenging yourself, the faster you'll see positive changes.

To measure your improvements, we recommend doing baseline tests of endurance, strength, and flexibility before you start your core program. Then retest yourself every two to four weeks. Celebrating even small successes will help to fuel your motivation and determination.

When performing the tests, only do as many reps, or hold for as many seconds, as you can manage with good form while following the tempo specified. If necessary, use the easier variation of the exercise for your baseline test. Jot down the answers in the spaces provided.

Of course, you can track your gains in informal ways, too. Are any tasks easier to accomplish? Does your back hurt less? Is your forehand, swimming stroke, or golf swing more powerful? Do your clothes fit better? Are you standing up straighter? Has your balance improved? Factors like these will help you gauge your improvement over time, perhaps even more meaningfully than being able to do a certain number of reps or sets.

Endurance

Perform a front plank (see page 24), holding it for as long as you can.

Date of baseline: _____ How many seconds _____
   Date of test 1: _____ How many seconds _____
   Date of test 2: _____ How many seconds _____
   Date of test 3: _____ How many seconds _____
   Date of test 4: _____ How many seconds _____

Strength

Perform the plié exercise (see page 19), doing as many reps as you can.

Date of baseline: _____ How many reps _____
   Date of test 1: _____ How many reps _____
   Date of test 2: _____ How many reps _____
   Date of test 3: _____ How many reps _____
   Date of test 4: _____ How many reps _____

Flexibility

Perform the YMCA sit-and-reach test (described below) three times, noting the best measurement. Have a friend help you keep your legs straight as you reach without interfering with your movement, and check the measurements. If you don't have a yardstick, simply note how far the tips of your fingers extend beyond a body landmark like your knees, ankles, or toes.

Starting position. Tape a yardstick to the floor by running a strip of tape across the 15-inch mark. After a full-body warm-up lasting at least five minutes, take off your shoes and sit on the floor with your legs 10 to 12 inches apart. Position yourself so that the yardstick is between your legs, with the zero mark pointing toward you and your heels at the 15-inch mark.

Movement. Put one hand on top of the other,

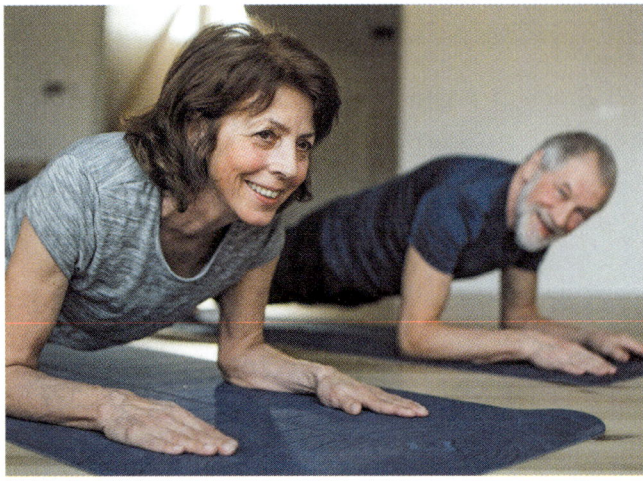

You can chart your progress on core exercises by keeping track of some simple measures—for example, how many seconds you can hold a front plank or how long you can balance on one leg.

middle fingers touching. Exhale as you slowly stretch forward with arms extended and your fingertips sliding lightly along the yardstick (or floor, if there is no yardstick). Don't bounce or jerk. Return to the starting position. Rest a few seconds and repeat. Do three sit-and-reach stretches, noting the farthest measurement.

Date of baseline: _____ How far did you stretch? _____
   Date of test 1: _____ How far did you stretch? _____
   Date of test 2: _____ How far did you stretch? _____
   Date of test 3: _____ How far did you stretch? _____
   Date of test 4: _____ How far did you stretch? _____

Balance

Perform a single-leg stance. To do this, you start by standing comfortably near a wall, holding your arms in any position you choose. Lift one foot an inch or two off the floor so that you are balancing on the other foot. Time how long you can do this before having to put the raised foot down or touch the wall for support.

If you can't stand on one leg unassisted, lightly touch the wall or hold the back of a chair with one or both hands for support. Use less support as you improve your balance. If this exercise is too easy, try timing yourself while standing on a less stable surface, such as a Bosu, or as you bounce and catch a ball while you have one foot raised off the floor.

Date of baseline: _____ How many seconds _____
   Date of test 1: _____ How many seconds _____
   Date of test 2: _____ How many seconds _____
   Date of test 3: _____ How many seconds _____
   Date of test 4: _____ How many seconds _____

If you can hold a single-leg stance for 60 seconds or more, you have excellent balance. If you can't hold the stance for more than 10 seconds, you are at risk for a fall. In this case, talk to your doctor about ways to improve your balance and reduce your chances of falling.

Standing Core Workout

The Standing Core Workout is a great first step toward a stronger midsection (or a great second step, if you choose to begin with the Floor Core Workout). It allows you to practice classic movement patterns like squats and lunges on a stable surface, yet it also teaches you some new twists on the standard moves. Since it requires only body weight to help you build strength, it's a perfect routine for home or travel. Because you stand while doing the exercises in this workout, it's also easy to do a few moves throughout the day.

The routine includes seven moves that, together, work a number of core muscles, including the erector spinae, transversus abdominis, quadratus lumborum, rectus abdominis, and glutes. As you do the exercises, focus on good form. If you find any of these exercises especially difficult, do fewer reps or try the "Make it easier" variation. For a more vigorous workout, try the "Make it harder" version. Remember to begin with a short warm-up (see "Warm up," page 9).

Equipment (optional): Sturdy chair.

STANDING CORE WORKOUT

① Leg swing

Reps: 10 per leg
Sets: 1–3
Tempo: 3–3
Rest: 30–90 seconds between sets

Starting position: Stand up straight with your feet together and your hands on your hips.

Movement: Lift your right leg straight out to the side until your foot is about six inches off the floor. Then swing your leg to the left across your body. Lift it back out to the side for the next rep. Keep your hips evenly aligned throughout. Finish all reps, then repeat with the other leg. That's one set.

Tips and techniques:
- Keep your spine neutral and your shoulders down and back.
- Don't lean to the side.
- Tighten the buttock on your standing leg for stability as you swing the opposite leg.

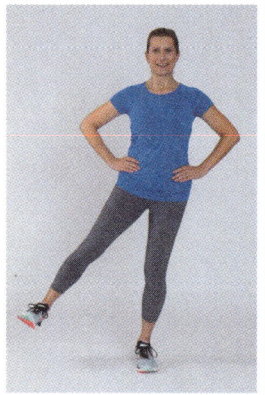 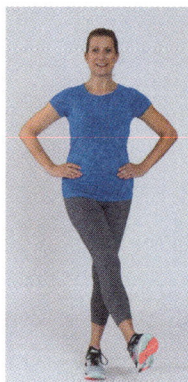

Make it easier: Hold on to a chair.
Make it harder: Hold the side leg lift for four counts before swinging your leg across your body.

② Diagonal knee pull

Reps: 10 per leg
Sets: 1–3
Tempo: 3–3
Rest: 30–90 seconds between sets

Starting position: Stand up straight, with your feet about shoulder-width apart and your arms extended overhead and slanting to the left.

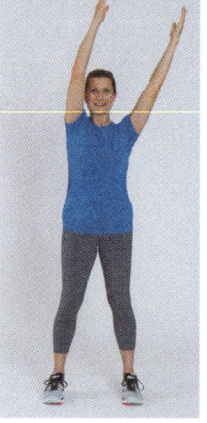 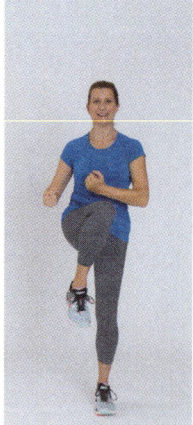

Movement: Pull your elbows down across your body, while lifting your right knee toward your left elbow. Return to the starting position. Finish all reps, then repeat with the left leg. That's one set.

Tips and techniques:
- Keep your chest lifted and your shoulders down and back.
- Tighten your abdominal muscles throughout.
- Tighten the buttock of your standing leg for stability.

Make it easier: Hold on to the back of a chair with one hand for support. Or do knee lifts only, keeping your hands on your hips or out to the sides.
Make it harder: Lift and lower your knee without your foot touching the floor in between, or lightly touching the floor with your toes only.

18   Core Exercises

STANDING CORE WORKOUT

3) Plié

Reps: 10
Sets: 1–3
Tempo: 3-1-3
Rest: 30–90 seconds between sets

Starting position: Stand up straight with your feet wider than your hips. Turn your toes slightly outward (rotating from the hips) and rest your hands on your thighs.

Movement: Keep your back straight as you bend your knees and lower your buttocks toward the floor. Stop before your buttocks reach knee level. Hold. Exhale as you return to the starting position.

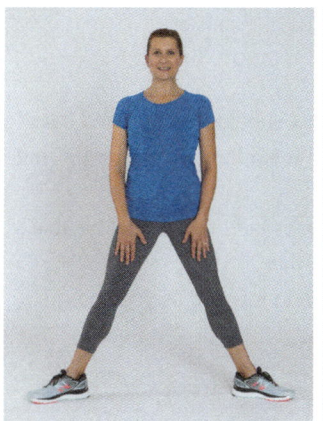 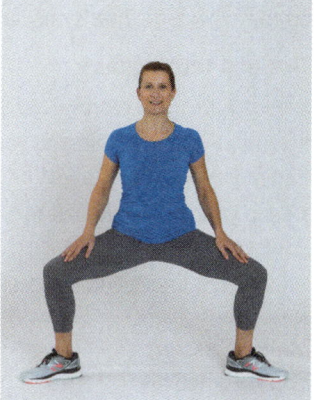

Tips and techniques:
- Lower your buttocks straight down toward the floor, not back and down as you do when squatting.
- Keep your knees aligned over your ankles when in the plié position.
- Keep your spine neutral, body upright, and shoulders down and back.
- Tighten abdominal muscles throughout and squeeze your glutes and inner thighs as you rise.

Make it easier: Make your pliés smaller. (Don't bend your knees as much.)
Make it harder: Hold the plié for four counts before returning to the starting position.

4) Alternating reverse lunge

Reps: 10
Sets: 1–3
Tempo: 3-1-3
Rest: 30–90 seconds between sets

Starting position: Stand up straight with your feet together and your hands at your sides.

Movement: Step back onto the ball of your right foot and sink into a lunge, bending your knees and bringing your hands up in front of your chest, elbows bent. Hold. Your left knee should align over your left ankle, and your right knee should point to the floor. Exhale as you return to the starting position. Repeat with your left leg. This is one rep.

Tips and techniques:
- Keep your weight evenly distributed between the right and left feet.
- In the lunge position, your shoulder, hip, and rear knee should be aligned.
- Your front knee should be directly over your ankle.
- Don't lean forward or back.
- Keep your spine neutral and your shoulders down and back.

Make it easier: Make your lunge smaller by not lowering so far down. Or, do stationary lunges, starting with your feet apart and maintaining that position for all reps.
Make it harder: Hold the lunge for four counts before returning to the starting position. Or, raise your opposite arm overhead as you step back, and then lower it as you return to the starting position.

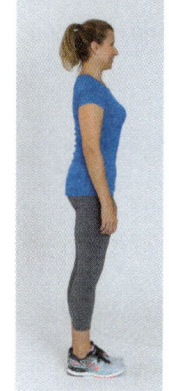 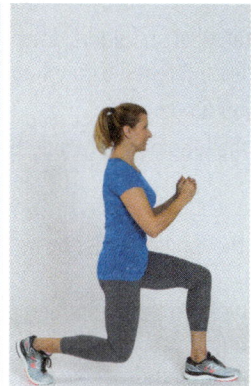 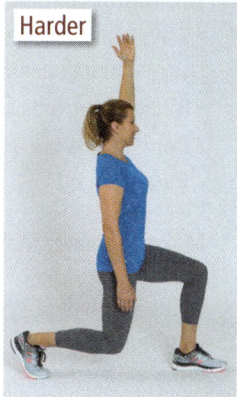

 **Special thanks to Michele Stanten,** the fitness consultant for this report, for demonstrating the exercises and stretches depicted here.

STANDING CORE WORKOUT

5) Side lunge

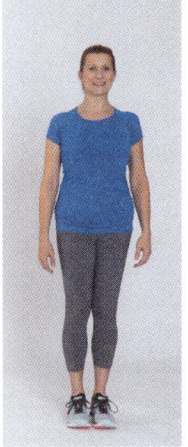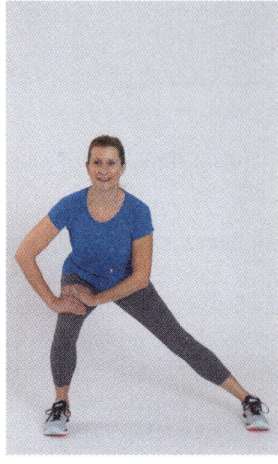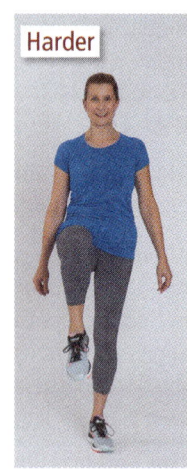
Harder

Reps: 10 per side
Sets: 1–3
Tempo: 3–1–3
Rest: 30–90 seconds between sets

Starting position: Stand up straight with your feet together and your hands at your sides.

Movement: Step way out to the side with your right foot, while keeping your left foot in place. As your right foot hits the ground, transfer most of your weight to your right leg, hinge forward at your hips, and bend your right knee, lowering into a lunge. Hold. Keep your left leg straight and put your hands on your right thigh for support. Exhale as you return to the starting position. Finish all reps, then repeat on the opposite side. That's one set.

Tips and techniques:
- Keep your spine neutral, your shoulders down and back, and your abdominal muscles tightened throughout.
- Hinge at the hips as you lunge.
- Don't let the knee of the lunging leg extend beyond your toes.

Make it easier: Make the lunge smaller by not lowering so far down.
Make it harder: As you return to the starting position, bring your right knee up in front of you, then immediately swing it out and lower into the next lunge.

6) Side squat with knee lift

Reps: 10 per side
Sets: 1–3
Tempo: 3–1–3
Rest: 30–90 seconds between sets

Starting position: Stand up straight with your feet together and your hands at your sides.

Movement: Step to the right, hinge forward at your hips, and bend your hips and knees to lower your buttocks into a squat as if sitting down. As you do so, clasp your hands loosely in front of your chest. Hold. Exhale as you lift up from the squat, and bring your right knee up and your hands to your sides. Return to the squat and repeat until you finish all reps. Repeat on the other side. That's one set.

Tips and techniques:
- Keep your spine neutral and your shoulders down and back.
- Bend at your hips, hinging your torso forward about 45°, but keep your head and chest lifted.
- Keep your knees aligned over your feet. You should be able to see your toes if you glance down.
- Keep your knees and toes pointing forward as you squat.

Make it easier: Skip the knee lift.
Make it harder: Hold each squat for four counts before rising up from the squat for the knee lift.

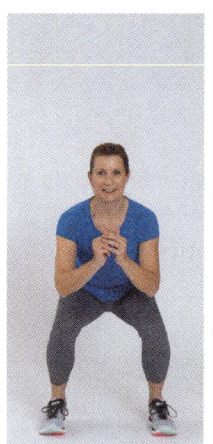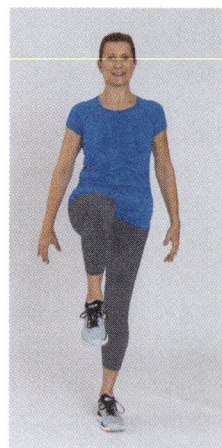

STANDING CORE WORKOUT

7 Curtsy lunge

Reps: 10 per side
Sets: 1–3
Tempo: 3–1–3
Rest: 30–90 seconds between sets

Starting position: Stand up straight with your right leg out to your side, toes touching the floor. Place your hands on your hips.

Movement: Bring your right foot behind your left leg. Place your weight on the ball of the rear foot and bend your knees as if curtsying. Hold. Exhale as you return to the starting position. Finish all reps, then repeat the sequence on the opposite side. That's one set.

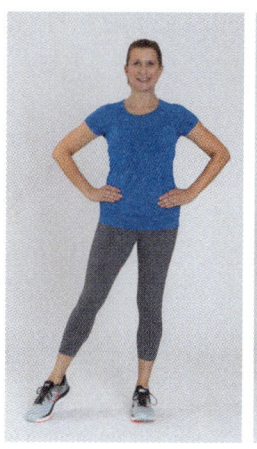
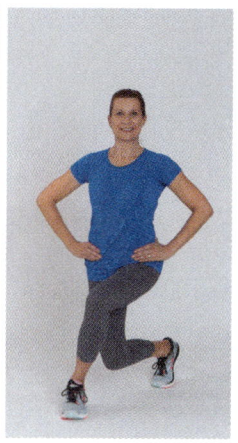
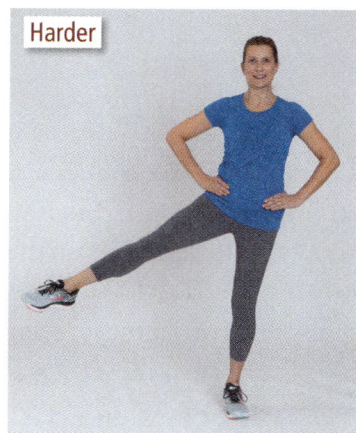

Tips and techniques:
- Keep your spine neutral and your shoulders down and back.
- Keep your weight evenly distributed between the front and back feet when you are in the curtsy position.
- When returning to the starting position, exhale and tighten the buttock on your standing leg for stability as you lift up.

Make it easier: Make the curtsy smaller.
Make it harder: Rise from the curtsy, then lift your leg out to the side before returning to the starting position.

 **You're not done yet** See "Finish with stretches," page 43, for a set of seven stretches to end your routine. Stretching helps to prevent stiffness and preserve flexibility and range of motion.

www.health.harvard.edu   Core Exercises   21

Floor Core Workout

If you started with the Standing Core Workout, the Floor Core Workout is a great next step toward a stronger midsection. But if you have balance issues or simply prefer exercises on the floor, you can start with this routine. The Floor Core Workout allows you to practice essential movements like bridges and planks on a stable surface, yet it also teaches you some new twists on those standard exercises. It requires no special equipment other than your own body weight to help you build strength, making it perfect for home or travel. However, you may want a mat for comfort.

As you do the exercises, focus on good form. If you find any of these exercises especially difficult, do fewer reps or try the "Make it easier" variation. For a more vigorous workout, try the "Make it harder" variation. Remember to begin with a short warm-up (see "Warm up," page 9).

Equipment: Mat or carpet for comfort.

FLOOR CORE WORKOUT

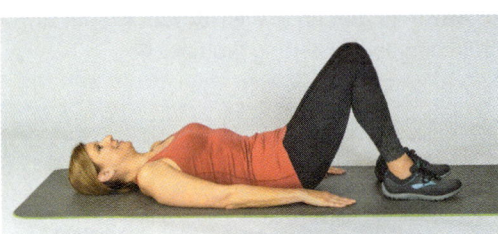
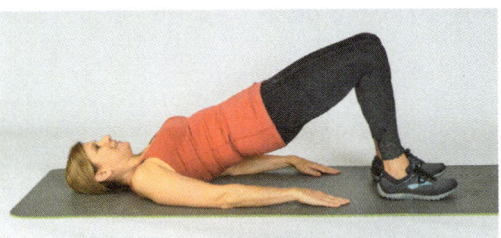
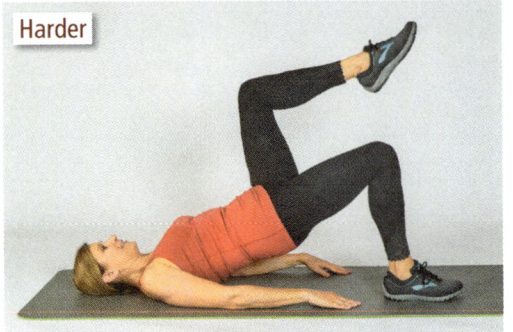
Harder

1 Bridge

Reps: 10
Sets: 1–3
Tempo: 3–1–3
Rest: 30–90 seconds between sets

Starting position: Lie on your back with your knees bent and feet flat on the floor, hip-width apart. Place your arms at your sides. Relax your shoulders against the floor.

Movement: Tighten your buttocks, then lift your hips up off the floor until they form a straight line with your hips and shoulders. Hold. Return to the starting position.

Tips and techniques:
• Tighten your buttocks before lifting.
• Keep your shoulders, hips, knees, and feet evenly aligned.
• Keep your shoulders down and relaxed into the floor.

Make it easier: Lift your buttocks just slightly off the floor.
Make it harder: Lift up into the bridge to a count of two. Pull your left knee in toward your chest, keeping your pelvis level. Hold for two counts, then return to the bridge to a count of two. Pull your right knee in toward your chest. Hold for two counts, then return to the bridge to a count of two. Lower your buttocks to the floor. This is one rep.

22   Core Exercises   www.health.harvard.edu

FLOOR CORE WORKOUT

② Clam

Reps: 10 per side
Sets: 1–3
Tempo: 3-1-3
Rest: 30–90 seconds between sets

Starting position: Lie on your right side, knees bent and heels in line with your buttocks. Rest your head on your right arm and place your left hand on the floor in front of you.

Movement: Engage your glutes and lift your left knee up toward the ceiling, while keeping your feet together. Hold. Then slowly lower to the starting position. Finish all reps, then repeat on the opposite side. That's one set.

Tips and techniques:
• Keep your hips stacked and still throughout the movement.
• You don't have to lift the top knee high.
• Think about rotating your femur (thighbone) while keeping your pelvis stable. If you feel it in your glutes, you're doing it correctly.

Make it easier: Don't lift your top knee as high.
Make it harder: Hold the knee lift for a count of three.

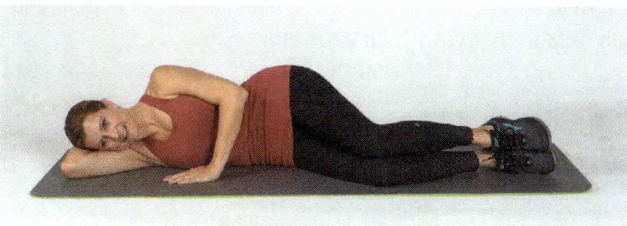

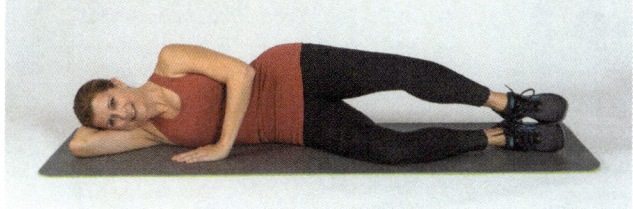

③ Alternating toe taps

Reps: 10
Sets: 1–3
Tempo: 3-1-3
Rest: 30–90 seconds between sets

Starting position: Lie on your back. Raise your knees so that they are aligned over your hips, with your legs forming 90° angles at the knees and your shins parallel to the floor. Rest your hands at your sides.

Movement: Tighten your abdominal muscles, maintaining a neutral spine. Keeping your knees bent and your left leg stationary, lower your right leg and tap your right foot on the floor. Hold. Then raise your right leg back to the starting position. Repeat with your left leg. This is one rep.

Tips and techniques:
• Keep your spine neutral throughout.
• Lower the foot only as far as you comfortably can while maintaining a neutral spine.
• Breathe comfortably throughout, exhaling as you lower the foot toward the floor.

Make it easier: Lower each foot less.
Make it harder: Lower both feet toward the floor simultaneously while keeping your spine neutral.

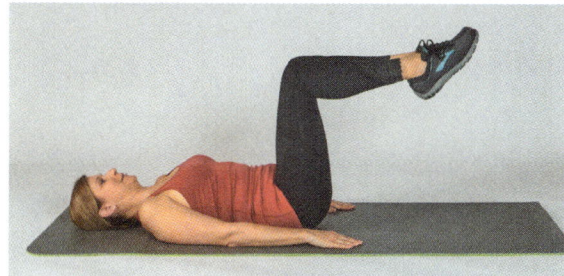

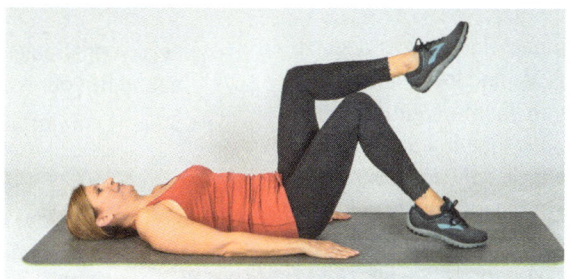

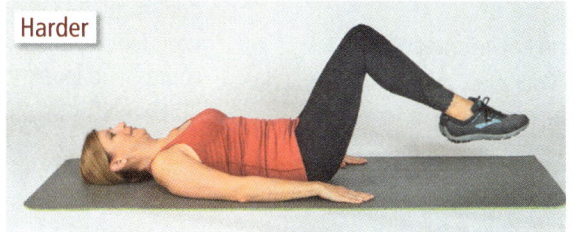

Harder

www.health.harvard.edu   Core Exercises

FLOOR CORE WORKOUT

4 Opposite arm and leg raise

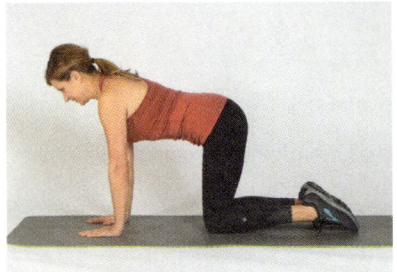
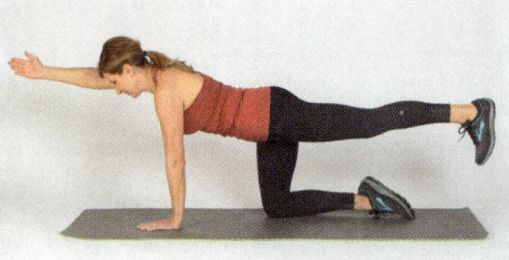
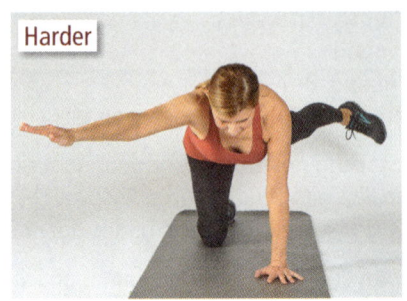

Harder

Reps: 10
Sets: 1–3
Tempo: 3–1–3
Rest: 30–90 seconds between sets

Starting position: Kneel on all fours with your hands and knees directly aligned under your shoulders and hips. Keep your head and spine neutral.

Movement: Extend your left leg off the floor behind you while reaching out in front of you with your right arm. Keeping your hips and shoulders squared, try to bring that leg and arm parallel to the floor. Hold. Return to the starting position, then repeat with your right leg and left arm. This is one rep.

Tips and techniques:
- Keep your shoulders and hips squared to maintain alignment throughout.
- Keep your head and spine neutral.
- Think of pulling your hand and leg in opposite directions, lengthening your torso.

Make it easier: Extend your right arm; return to the starting position. Extend your left leg; return to the starting position. Repeat with the left arm, followed by the right leg. This is one rep.
Make it harder: Move your extended arm and leg on a diagonal (think of a clock: instead of noon and 6, move them to 2 and 8, or 10 and 4, depending on which arm and leg are in action) and then back to the center before lowering.

5 Front plank

Reps: 2–4
Sets: 1
Hold: 15–60 seconds
Rest: 30–90 seconds between reps

Starting position: Start on your hands and knees.

Movement: Tighten your abdominal muscles and lower your upper body onto your forearms, clasping your hands together and aligning your shoulders directly over your elbows. Extend both legs with your feet flexed and toes touching the floor so that you balance your body in a line like a plank. Hold.

Tips and techniques:
- Keep your neck and spine neutral during the plank.
- Don't bend at your hips.
- Don't drop your belly toward the floor.
- Don't drop your head.

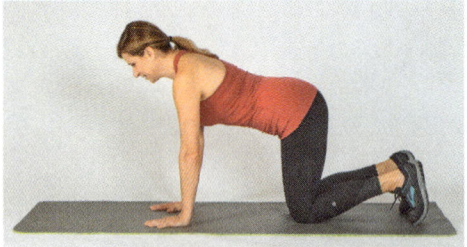
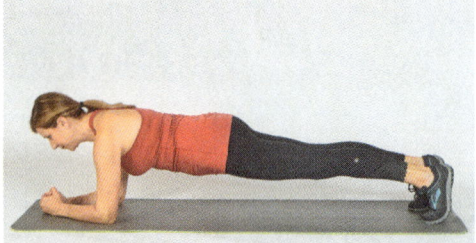

- Keep your shoulders down and back, not up by your ears.
- Breathe comfortably.

Make it easier: Instead of extending your legs, put your knees on the floor for a modified plank position.
Make it harder: While holding your body in the plank position, lift your right foot off the floor, hold for eight counts, and lower it to the floor. Then lift your left foot, hold for eight counts, and lower it to the floor. Continue doing this for 15 to 60 seconds.

Easier
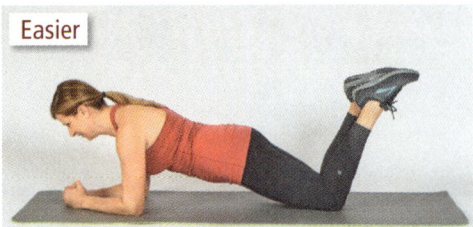

Harder
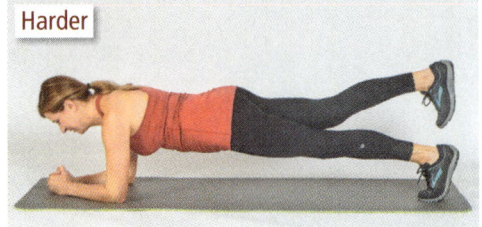

FLOOR CORE WORKOUT

6 Side plank

Reps: 2–4 per side
Sets: 1
Hold: 15–60 seconds
Rest: 30–90 seconds between reps

Starting position: Lie in a straight line on your right side. Support your upper body on your right forearm with your shoulder aligned directly over your elbow. Stack your left foot on top of your right foot. Rest your left hand on your left hip.

Movement: Tighten your abdominal muscles. Exhale as you lift your hips off the floor and raise your left arm toward the ceiling. Keeping shoulders and hips in a straight line, balance on your right forearm. Hold. Return to the starting position. Finish all reps, then repeat lying on your left side. That's one set.

Tips and techniques:
- Keep your head and spine neutral, and align your shoulder over your elbow.
- Focus on lifting the bottom hip.
- Keep your shoulders down and back.

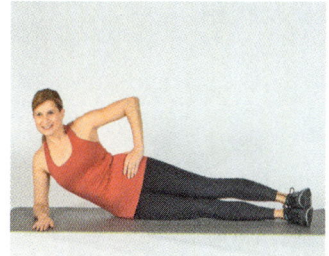
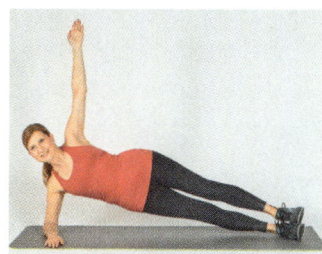
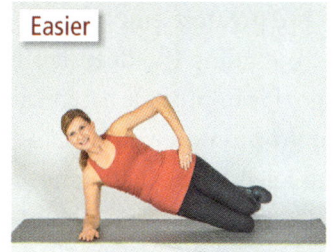 Easier
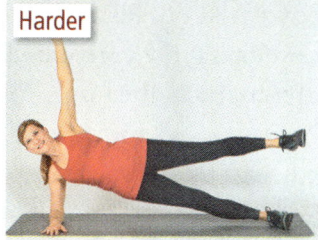 Harder

Make it easier: Bend at your knees and put your feet behind you. Keep your knees on the floor as you lift your hips.
Make it harder: Lift your top foot up toward the ceiling.

---

7 Front plank with knee drop

Reps: 10
Sets: 1–3
Tempo: 2–2
Rest: 30–90 seconds between sets

Starting position: Get down on all fours with your hands and knees directly aligned under your shoulders and hips, respectively. Extend both legs with your feet flexed and toes touching the floor so that you balance your body in a line as you would in a front plank (see page 24), but with your weight resting on your hands rather than your elbows.

Movement: Tighten your abdominal muscles. Lower both knees toward the floor without touching it, then extend your legs again to return to the plank position. This is one rep.

Tips and techniques:
- Keep your neck and spine neutral during the plank.
- Keep your shoulders down and back.
- Breathe comfortably.

Make it easier: Reduce the number of reps in each set to 3–5. You can gradually work up to 10.
Make it harder: This variation is a two-part movement, starting from the plank position. First, bring your left knee toward your left shoulder, then return to the plank position. Second, bring your right knee toward your right shoulder, then return to the plank position. Do this five times.

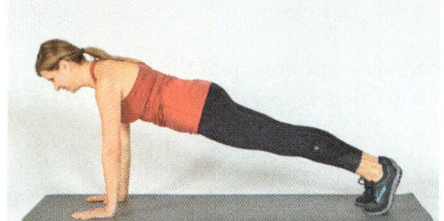
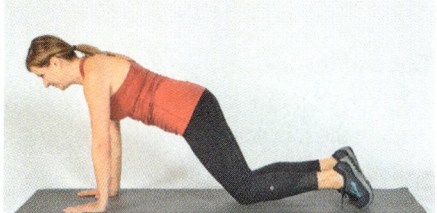
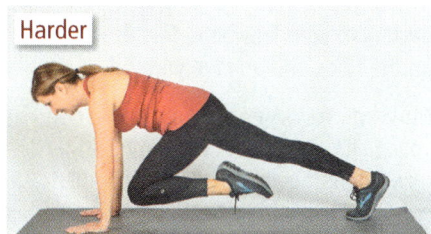 Harder

>>> **You're not done yet** See "Finish with stretches," page 43, for a set of seven stretches to end your routine. Stretching helps to prevent stiffness and preserve flexibility and range of motion.

www.health.harvard.edu   Core Exercises   25

Pilates Workout

The Pilates Workout is a great next step after mastering either the Standing Core Workout or the Floor Core Workout. Of the many types of exercise you could do, Pilates places the greatest emphasis on developing the core muscles, including the deep layer of muscles in the torso. The goal is to provide a central "powerhouse" for movement, to promote smooth and efficient motion by helping to keep the body balanced and aligned, and to support a healthy spine. Pilates also enhances proprioception (awareness of your body in space) and control of movements.

There are two main types of Pilates classes—apparatus and mat. The former requires specialized equipment (including a machine called a reformer), so we focus here on a selection of mat exercises that don't require anything special. You'll be doing fewer reps during this routine, because quality is more important than quantity. You want to concentrate on executing the moves with proper alignment and precision to maximize results.

Throughout, try to focus on keeping your core muscles tight—or as instructors sometimes put it, tightening your "inner corset"—in order to keep your pelvis, shoulders, and other parts of the body steady during an exercise. To use the analogy cited earlier in this report, it's like pulling in your muscles to zip up a tight jacket and pair of jeans. Tightening the core muscles, however, does not mean keeping your spine rigid all the time. Pilates emphasizes the importance of spinal articulation—or the ability to isolate spinal movements one vertebra at a time. A good illustration of this is the pelvic curl exercise, below. To see how the motion rolls through the spine, watch the video at www.health.harvard.edu/pelvic-curl.

If you find an exercise especially difficult, do fewer reps or try the "Make it easier" variation. For a more vigorous workout, try the "Make it harder" variation. Remember to begin with a short warm-up (see "Warm up," page 9).

Equipment: Mat or carpet for comfort.

PILATES WORKOUT

1 Pelvic curl

Reps: 5–7
Sets: 1–3
Tempo: 3–1–3
Rest: 30–90 seconds between sets

Starting position: Lie on your back with your legs bent, feet flat on the floor, and arms at your sides.

Movement: Contract your abs and curl your tailbone upward. Continue to roll upward, lifting your buttocks first, then your low and middle back, one vertebra at a time, until you are in a bridge position. Hold. Slowly roll back down to the starting position.

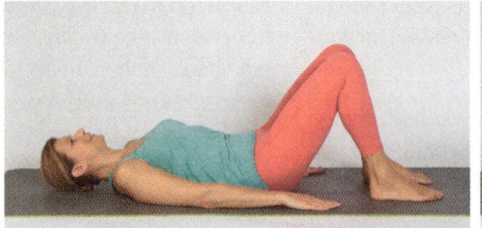

Tips and techniques:
- Tighten your core muscles before executing the movement.
- Lift until your body is in a straight line from your knees to your shoulders, no higher.
- Don't let your knees fall out to the sides.

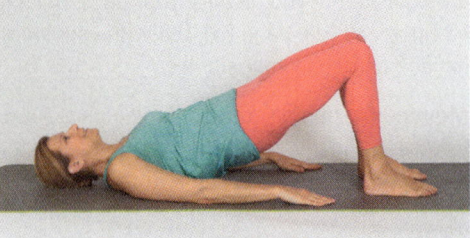

For a demonstration of this exercise, go to www.health.harvard.edu/pelvic-curl.

Make it easier: Do pelvic curls without lifting your back off the floor.
Make it harder: Hold for four counts before lowering.

PILATES WORKOUT

2) The hundred

Reps: 100
Sets: 1
Tempo: 1–1
Rest: 30–90 seconds between reps, if needed

Starting position: Lie on your back with your feet off the floor and hips and knees bent at 90°. Place your arms at your sides, palms down. Contract your abs and lift your head, shoulders, and arms off the floor.

Movement: Pump your arms up and down about four to six inches as you take five short breaths in and then five short breaths out. Without pausing in between, do this sequence a total of 10 times (a total of 100 arm pumps).

Tips and techniques:
- Tighten your core muscles before executing the movement.
- Keep your chin level, not tucked or pointing forward or upward. You should be able to fit your fist between your chin and your chest.
- Keep your shoulders and neck relaxed.

Make it easier: Keep your feet on the floor. Do fewer reps.
Make it harder: Extend your legs so they are at about a 45° angle to the floor.

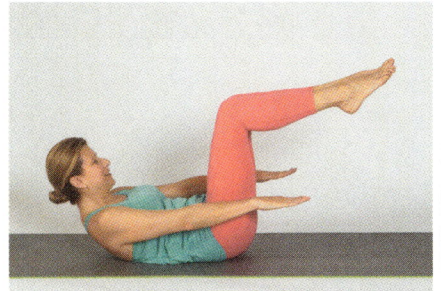
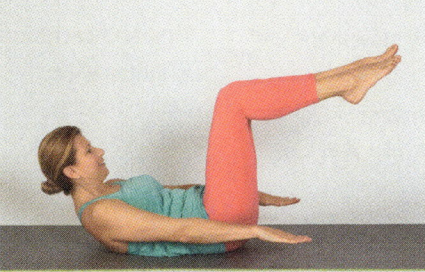
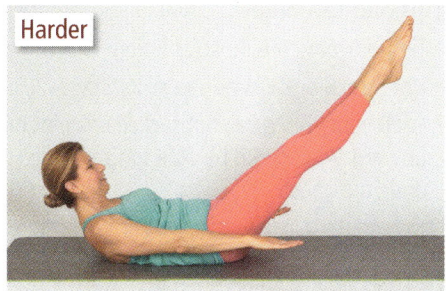

Harder

3) Single-leg circle

Reps: 5 in each direction per leg
Sets: 1–3
Tempo: 3 (more for bigger circles, less for smaller ones)
Rest: 30–90 seconds between sets

Starting position: Lie on your back with your legs bent and feet on the floor, arms at your sides, palms down. Extend your left leg straight up toward the ceiling, toes pointed.

Movement: Rotating from the hip only, draw five circles with your toes, out to the side, away from you, and then back to the starting position. Focus on stabilizing your pelvis and core, so that only your leg is moving. With the same leg, draw five more circles going the other direction. Repeat the sequence with your right leg. That's one set.

Tips and techniques:
- Tighten your core muscles before executing the movement.
- Keep your lower back on the floor.
- Your pelvis should remain still. If it isn't, make smaller circles.

Make it easier: Make smaller circles.
Make it harder: Make larger circles.

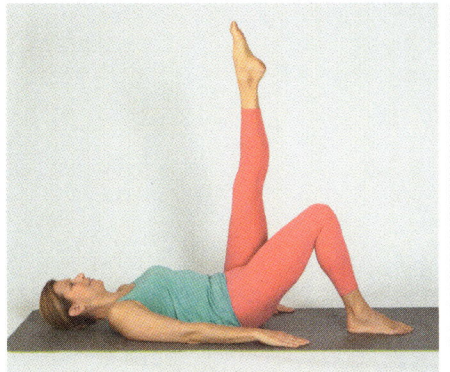
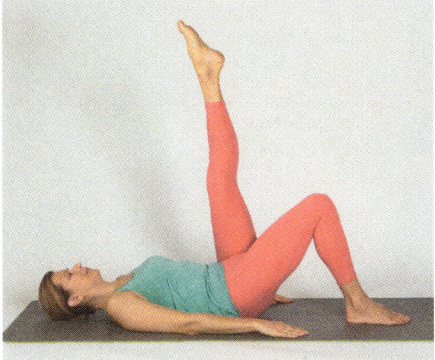
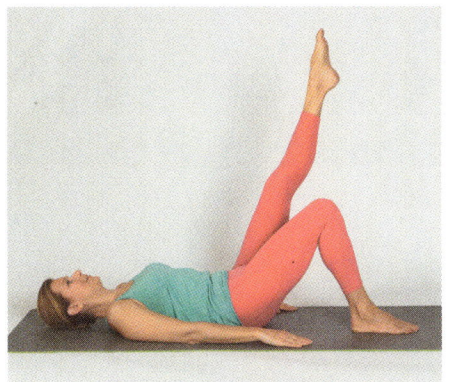

www.health.harvard.edu

PILATES WORKOUT

④ Single-leg stretch

Reps: 5–7
Sets: 1–3
Tempo: 3–1–3
Rest: 30–90 seconds between sets

Starting position: Lie on your back with your feet off the floor and your legs bent at 90°. Curl your head and shoulders off the floor and place your hands gently on the backs of your thighs.

Movement: Draw your right knee in toward your chest, gently grasping it with both hands. Simultaneously, extend your left leg at a 45° angle to the floor. Hold. Switch legs, drawing your left knee in toward your chest and extending your right leg. That's one rep.

Tips and techniques:
- Tighten your core muscles before executing the movement.
- Don't rock or twist as you switch legs.
- Keep your chin level, not tucked or pointing forward or upward. You should be able to fit your fist between your chin and your chest.

Make it easier: Extend your leg higher up toward the ceiling. Or, keep your head on the mat.
Make it harder: Extend your leg closer to the floor.

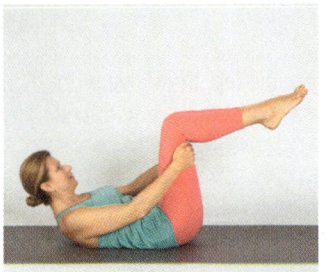
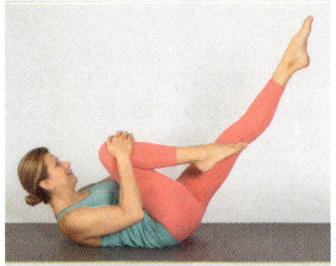
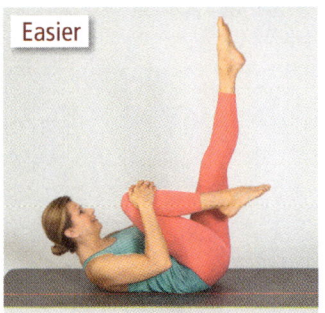
Easier
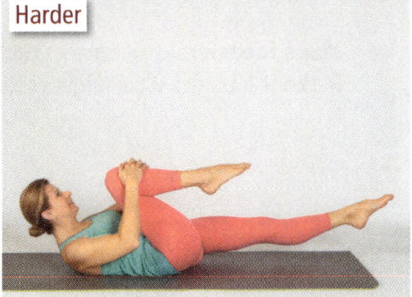
Harder

⑤ Double-leg stretch

Reps: 5–7
Sets: 1–3
Tempo: 3–1–3
Rest: 30–90 seconds between sets

Starting position: Lie on your back with your feet off the floor and your legs bent at 90°. Curl your head and shoulders off the floor and extend your arms toward your lower legs.

Movement: Extend your legs at a 45° angle to the floor as you reach with your arms overhead. Hold. Return to the starting position.

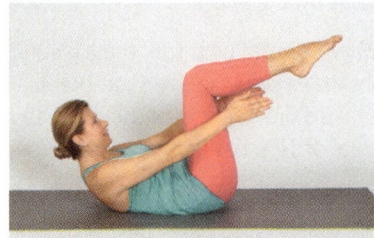

Tips and techniques:
- Tighten your core muscles before executing the movement.
- Keep your chin level, not tucked or pointing forward or upward. You should be able to fit your fist between your chin and your chest.
- Keep your shoulders and neck relaxed.

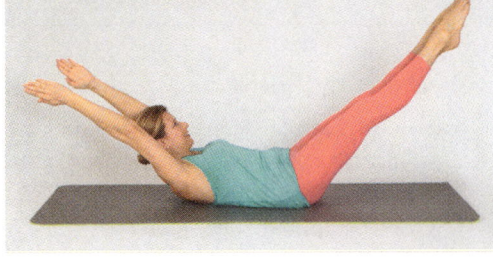

Make it easier: Extend your legs higher up toward the ceiling. Or, keep your head on the mat.
Make it harder: Extend your legs closer to the floor.

PILATES WORKOUT

6 Side-lying kick front and back

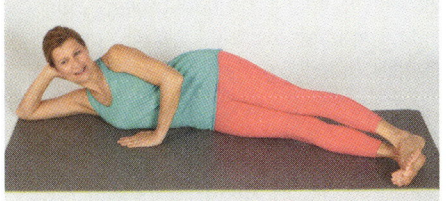
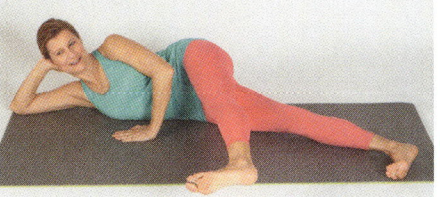
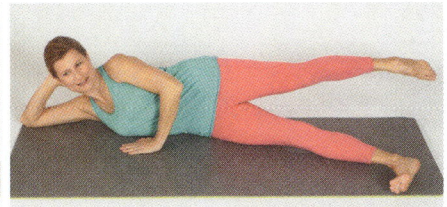

Reps: 5–7 per leg
Sets: 1–3
Tempo: 3–3
Rest: 30–90 seconds between sets

Starting position: Lie on your right side with your legs on a diagonal in front of you and your feet flexed. Support your head with your right arm and hand, and place your left hand on the floor in front of you.

Movement: Swing your left leg in front of you as far as is comfortable without moving the rest of your body. Then point your left foot and sweep your leg back behind you, only as far as you can without moving the rest of your body. This is one rep. Complete all reps, then repeat on the other side. That's one set.

Tips and techniques:
- Tighten your core muscles before executing the movement.
- Keep hips stacked vertically.
- Don't arch your back as you swing your leg behind you.
- Keep your hips and pelvis still. If you notice your upper body or hips rocking, don't kick so far.

Make it easier: Shorten the range of motion, not swinging your leg as far in front of you and behind you.
Make it harder: Support your body on your right knee and hand for left-leg kicks, and then switch sides.

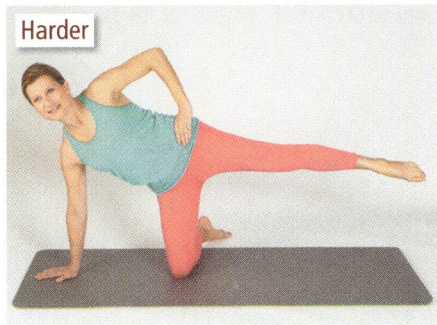

Harder

7 Side-lying double-leg lift

Reps: 5–7 per side
Sets: 1–3
Tempo: 3-1-3
Rest: 30–90 seconds between sets

Starting position: Lie on your right side with your toes pointed, your head lifted and supported on your bent right arm and hand, and your left hand on the floor in front of you.

Movement: Keeping your legs together, contract your abdominal muscles and raise your legs a few inches off the floor. Hold. Slowly lower. Finish all reps, then repeat lying on your left side. That's one set.

Tips and techniques:
- Tighten your core muscles before executing the movement.
- Keep your hips stacked vertically.
- Don't let your upper body roll forward or back as you lift.
- Squeeze your inner thighs together as you lift.

Make it easier: Bring your legs more in front of you for the starting position.
Make it harder: Hold your legs up for a count of three or four.

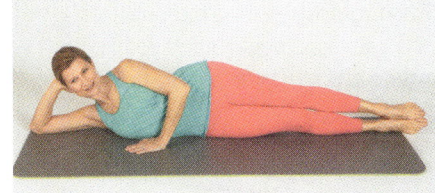
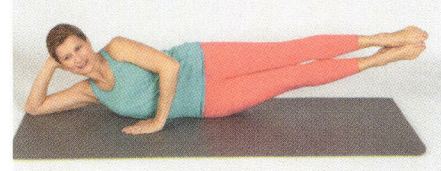
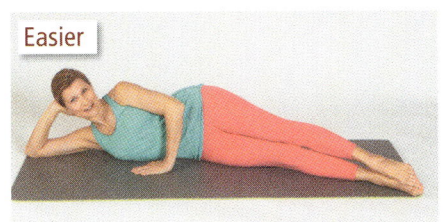

Easier

www.health.harvard.edu   Core Exercises 29

PILATES WORKOUT

8 Criss-cross

Reps: 8–10
Sets: 1–3
Tempo: 3–1–3
Rest: 30–90 seconds between sets

Starting position: Lie on your back with your feet off the floor and your legs bent at 90°. Place your hands lightly behind your head, elbows pointing out to the sides. Contract your abs, raising your head and shoulders off the floor.

Movement: Bring your left shoulder and elbow toward your right knee, while extending your left leg. Hold. Switch sides, bringing your right shoulder and elbow toward your left knee. That's one rep.

Tips and techniques:
- Tighten your core muscles before executing the movement.
- Don't pull on your neck.
- Keep a fist-width distance between your chin and chest.
- Keep your hips and pelvis stable as you twist; don't rock.

Make it easier: Place your feet on the floor with your legs bent and perform the exercise using only your upper body.
Make it harder: Lower your extended leg closer to the floor.

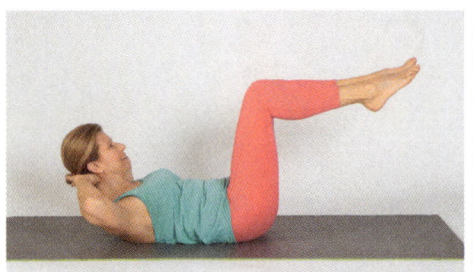
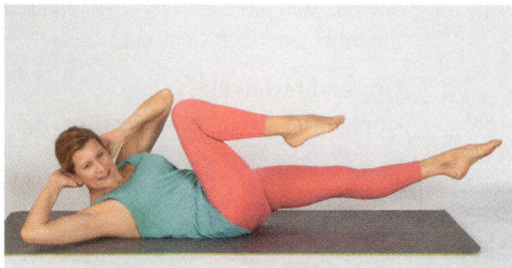

9 Letter T

Reps: 5–7
Sets: 1–3
Tempo: 3–1–3
Rest: 30–90 seconds between sets

Starting position: Lie facedown with your legs together and your arms extended out to your sides, palms down.

Movement: Raise your chest and head a few inches off the floor as you sweep your arms back alongside your body. Hold. Slowly lower back to the starting position.

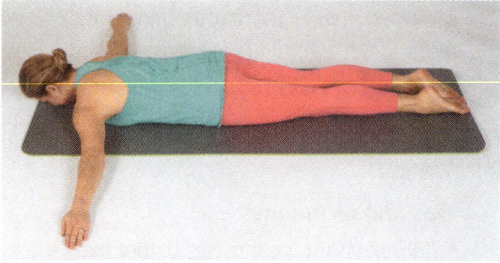
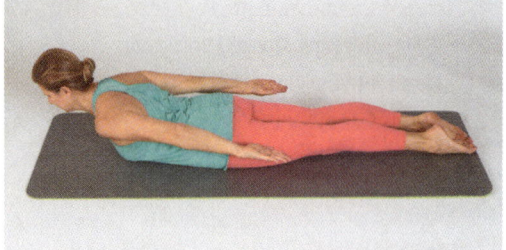

Tips and techniques:
- Keep a neutral neck, with your head in line with your spine.
- Don't look up, but keep your eyes on the floor.
- Press your legs into the mat as you lift.

Make it easier: Keep your arms by your sides as you lift and lower.
Make it harder: Hold the elevated position for a count of four.

>>> **You're not done yet** See "Finish with stretches," page 43, for a set of seven stretches to end your routine. Stretching helps to prevent stiffness and preserve flexibility and range of motion.

Core Exercises   www.health.harvard.edu

Medicine Ball Workout

After mastering essential movement patterns on a stable surface, as you did in any of the previous three workouts, you're ready to add a new challenge. Bumping up resistance with a weighted ball called a medicine ball makes your core muscles work harder. Start with a 4-pound ball (or lighter if needed), then work up to heavier balls over time, as the exercises become easier to do. The rotational and diagonal moves in this workout tone the waist and are a great tune-up for people who enjoy racquet sports, golf, and swimming.

Focus on good form. If you find an exercise especially difficult, do fewer reps or try the "Make it easier" variation. For a more vigorous workout, try the "Make it harder" variation. Remember to begin with a short warm-up (see "Warm up," page 9).

Equipment: Medicine ball; mat or carpet for comfort.

MEDICINE BALL WORKOUT

1 Cross chop and lift

Reps: 10 per side
Sets: 1–3
Tempo: 2–1–2
Rest: 30–90 seconds between sets

Starting position: Holding a medicine ball, squat slightly with your feet hip-width apart, hinging at the hips and bending your knees. Position the medicine ball toward the outside of your left knee.

Movement: Keeping your arms extended, shift your body weight to your right foot, raising your left heel slightly as you stand and lift the medicine ball diagonally up over your right shoulder. Hold. In a chopping motion, bring the medicine ball down and across your body, shifting back to the starting position. Finish all reps, then repeat on the other side. That's one set.

Tips and techniques:
- Keep your spine neutral and your shoulders down and back.
- Reach only as far as is comfortable.

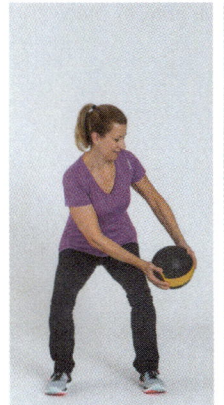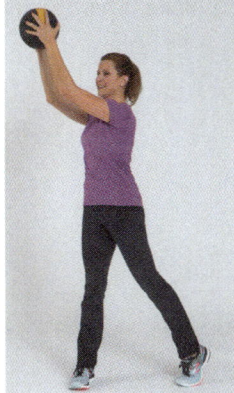

- Hinge at the hips and bend your knees slightly as you reach down.

Make it easier: Do the exercise without a medicine ball.
Make it harder: Use a heavier medicine ball.

2 Plié with overhead lift

Reps: 10
Sets: 1–3
Tempo: 3–1–3
Rest: 30–90 seconds between sets

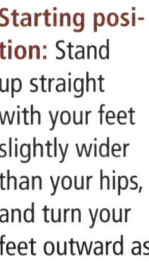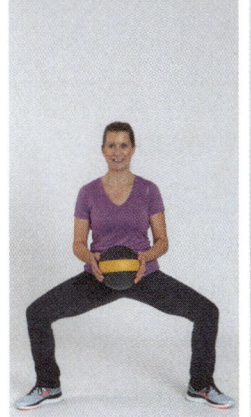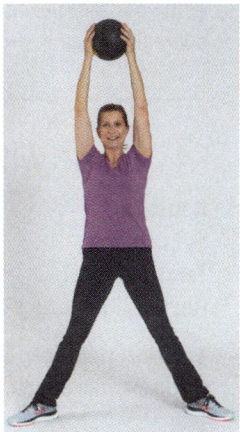

Starting position: Stand up straight with your feet slightly wider than your hips, and turn your feet outward as far as is comfortable. Hold the medicine ball at your waist.

Movement: Keeping your shoulders down and back, bend your knees until they are directly over your ankles. Hold. As you return to the starting position, lift the medicine ball overhead. Then for the remaining reps, lower the medicine ball below your waist as you sink into the plié.

Tips and techniques:
- Keep your torso upright and your spine neutral throughout.
- Keep your knees aligned with your toes.
- Tighten your inner thighs and glutes as you straighten your legs to return to the starting position.

Make it easier: Do the plié and lift without a medicine ball.
Make it harder: Use a heavier medicine ball.

MEDICINE BALL WORKOUT

③ Front plank on medicine ball

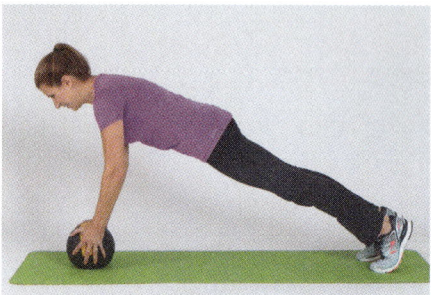
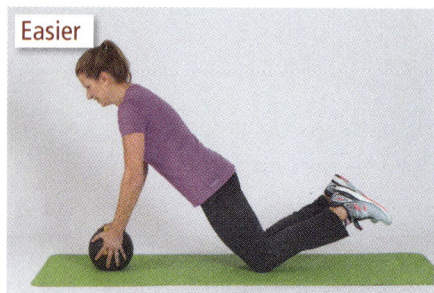
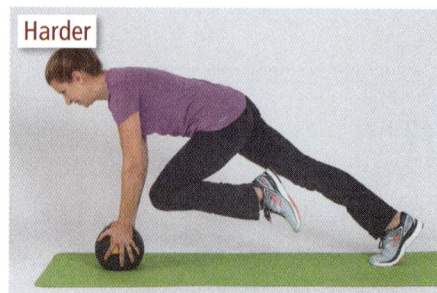

Reps: 2–4
Sets: 1
Hold: 15–60 seconds
Rest: 30–90 seconds between reps

Starting position: Start on your hands and knees with both hands gripping the sides of a medicine ball. Lift your chest and roll your shoulders down and back.

Movement: Tighten your abdominal muscles. Extend both legs with your feet flexed and toes on the floor so that your body is in a line like a plank. Hold.

Tips and techniques:
- Align your shoulders over your wrists.
- Keep your neck and spine neutral during the plank, not curving upward or downward.
- Keep your shoulders back and down, away from your ears.

Make it easier: Keep your knees on the floor. Be sure your body is in a straight line from head to knees.
Make it harder: While holding the plank, pull your left knee in toward your chest and then straighten it. Repeat with your right leg. That's one rep. Do 10 reps during a single plank.

④ Lunge with rotation

Reps: 10
Sets: 1–3
Tempo: 2–2–2–2
Rest: 30–90 seconds between sets

Starting position: Stand up straight, feet together, holding the medicine ball at your waist.

Movement: Step forward on your right leg, keeping the medicine ball in front of your torso as you bend your knees and sink into a lunge with your back knee pointing down toward the floor. Rotate your torso to the right as far as is comfortable, then come back to center. Step back to the starting position.

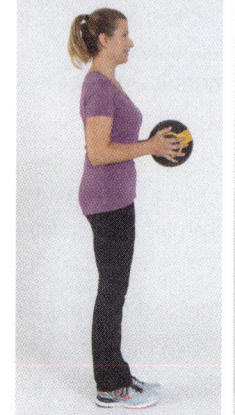
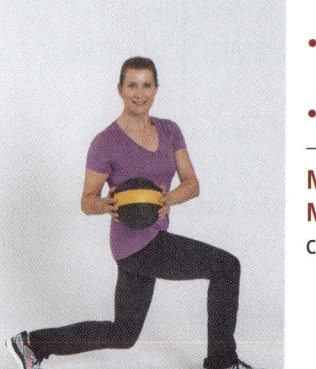

Repeat with your left leg forward, rotating your torso to the left. This completes one rep.

Tips and techniques:
- In the lunge position, your front knee should be directly over your ankle.
- The heel of your rear foot will come off the floor.
- Your back knee should be in line with your shoulder and hip before rotating.
- Keep your spine neutral throughout.

Make it easier: Skip the rotation.
Make it harder: Use a heavier medicine ball.

32   Core Exercises   www.health.harvard.edu

MEDICINE BALL WORKOUT

5) Overhead slam

Reps: 10
Sets: 1–3
Tempo: 1–1
Rest: 30–90 seconds between sets

Starting position: Stand tall with your feet about hip-width apart, toes pointing straight ahead. Hold a medicine ball with both hands at chest height, arms bent.

Movement: Extend your arms and bring the ball overhead. In a smooth motion, bring the ball down in front of you as you bend your hips and knees and throw the ball to the floor as hard as possible. Keep your arms straight. Catch the ball, or squat down to pick it up, and return to the starting position.

Tips and techniques:
- Keep your chest lifted.
- Don't bend at your waist.

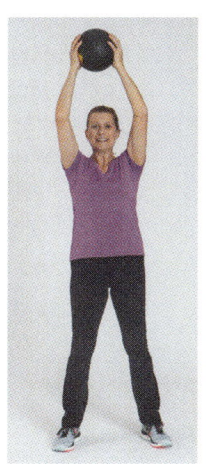 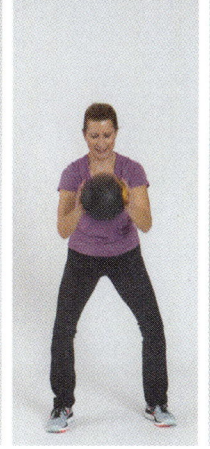 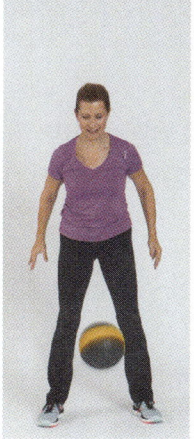 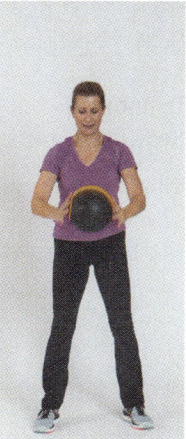

- Don't let your knees extend farther forward than your toes.

Make it easier: Instead of slamming the ball to the floor, simply let it drop.
Make it harder: Use a heavier medicine ball.

---

6) V-sit with twist

Reps: 10
Sets: 1–3
Tempo: 2–2–2–2
Rest: 30–90 seconds between sets

Starting position: Sit on the floor with your knees bent and feet flat on the floor, hip-width apart. Hold the medicine ball in front of your chest. Keep your chest lifted and your shoulders down and back. Lean back into a V position, bringing your feet off the floor with your knees bent and your lower legs parallel to the floor.

Movement: Rotate your torso to the right and bring the medicine ball toward your right hip, then return to center. Rotate to the left and bring the ball toward your left hip, then return to center. This completes one rep.

Tips and techniques:
- While holding the V position, keep your neck and spine neutral.
- As you rotate, keep your shoulders down and back, away from your ears.
- Breathe comfortably.

Make it easier: While in the V position, lower your heels or place them on the floor for support.
Make it harder: Use a heavier medicine ball.

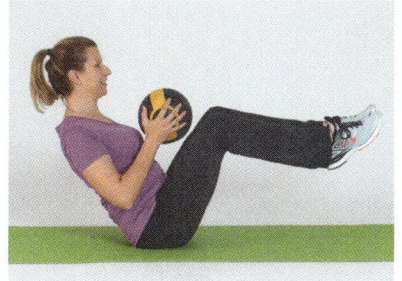 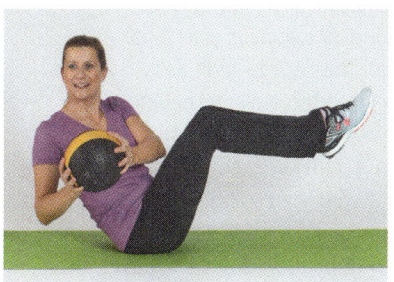

www.health.harvard.edu Core Exercises 33

MEDICINE BALL WORKOUT

7 Single-leg stance with medicine ball

Reps: 10 per side
Sets: 1–3
Tempo: 3–1–3
Rest: 30–90 seconds between sets

Starting position: Stand on your left leg with your right foot slightly behind you and lightly touching the floor. Hold the medicine ball at your waist.

Movement: Tighten your abdominal muscles and hinge forward at your hips, raising your right leg behind you and extending your arms to lower the medicine ball toward the floor. Be sure to keep your chest lifted and your shoulders down and back. Hold. Return to the starting position. Finish all reps, then repeat standing on your right leg. That's one set.

Tips and techniques:

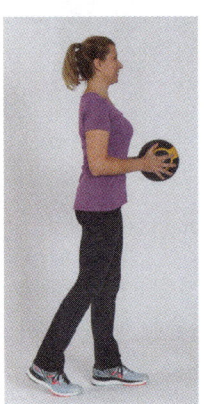 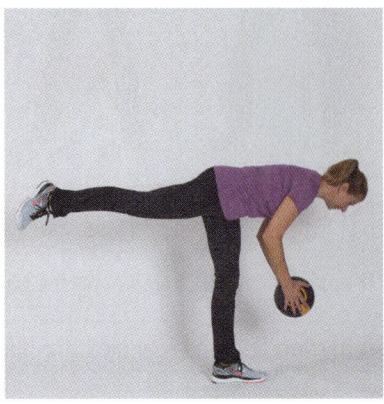 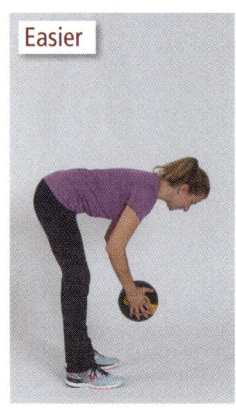

Easier

- Tighten the buttock of the standing leg for stability.
- Keep a slight bend in the knee of your standing leg.
- Lower the ball only as far as is comfortable.
- Exhale as you return to the starting position.

Make it easier: Keep both feet on the floor as you hinge forward at your hips, bending your knees slightly, and lower the ball toward the floor.
Make it harder: Use a heavier medicine ball.

8 Bridge with pullover

Reps: 10
Sets: 1–3
Tempo: 3–1–3
Rest: 30–90 seconds between sets

Starting position: Lie on your back with your knees bent and feet flat on the floor, hip-width apart, so that your heels are in line with your buttocks. Hold the medicine ball on the floor above your head.

Movement: Tighten your buttocks and lift your hips off the floor as high as is comfortable while keeping your spine neutral. Simultaneously lift the medicine ball up toward the ceiling above your chest. Hold. Lower your hips and the medicine ball to the starting position.

Tips and techniques:

- Keep your wrists, neck, and spine neutral throughout the movement.
- When lowering the medicine ball toward the floor, go only as far as is comfortable.
- Exhale as you lift your hips and the ball up off the floor.

Make it easier: Do the exercise without a medicine ball.
Make it harder: Use a heavier medicine ball.

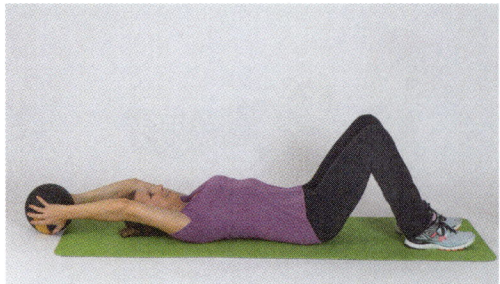 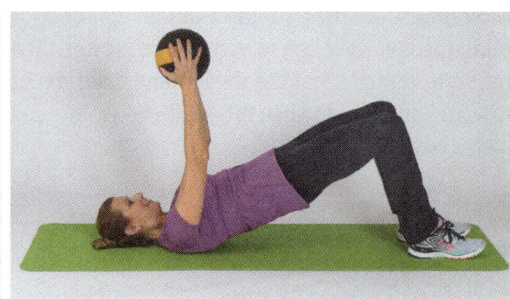

>>> **You're not done yet** See "Finish with stretches," page 43, for a set of seven stretches to end your routine. Stretching helps to prevent stiffness and preserve flexibility and range of motion.

34   Core Exercises   www.health.harvard.edu

Stability Ball Workout

Want a bigger bang for your exercise buck? After you've mastered essential movement patterns on a stable surface in any of the first three workouts, add a stability ball. By making a wide range of muscles—not just your core—work hard to hold a steady position and move your body smoothly through each step, these exercises improve your game in sports and daily activities.

Focus on good form. If you find an exercise especially difficult, do fewer reps or try the "Make it easier" variation. For a more vigorous workout, try the "Make it harder" variation.

Remember to begin with a short warm-up (see "Warm up," page 9).

Equipment: Stability ball; mat or carpet for comfort.

STABILITY BALL WORKOUT

1 Seated knee lift

Reps: 10 per side
Sets: 1–3
Tempo: 2–2
Rest: 30–90 seconds between sets

Starting position: Sit on the stability ball. Rest your hands at your sides on the ball.

Movement: Exhale as you lift your left knee and right hand straight toward the ceiling. Return to the starting position. Finish all reps, then repeat, lifting with your right knee and left hand. That's one set.

Tips and techniques:
- Keep your spine neutral and your shoulders down and back.
- Tighten your glutes to enhance stability.
- Focus on a spot in front of you to help you balance.

Make it easier: Hold the stability ball with both hands while lifting your knee.
Make it harder: Close your eyes.

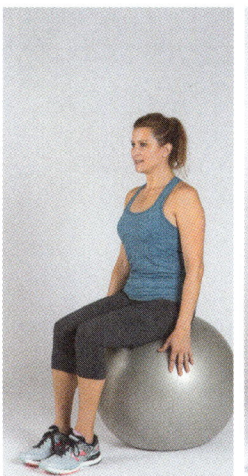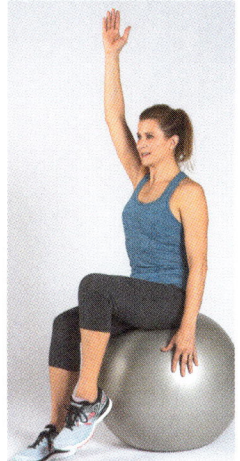

2 Twisting crunch on stability ball

Reps: 10
Sets: 1–3
Tempo: 3–1–3
Rest: 30–90 seconds between sets

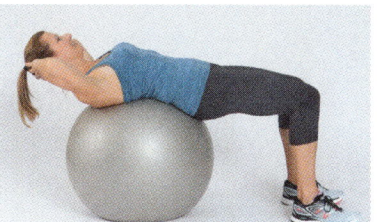

Starting position: Sit on the stability ball. Lean back and roll downward, walking your feet forward until the ball is centered under your back. Position your feet hip-width apart on the floor. Rest your hands lightly behind your head, elbows out.

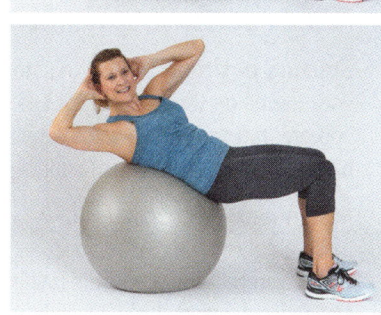

Movement: Tighten your abdominal muscles as you lift your head and shoulders up and then rotate to the right as if you're bringing your left elbow toward your right hip. Hold. Return to the starting position. Repeat, rotating to the left and bringing your right elbow across your body. That completes one rep.

Tips and techniques:
- Keep your spine neutral and your shoulders down and back.
- Keep your eyes focused on the ceiling in front of you as you lift.
- Between sets, sit on the ball. Clasp your hands and reach them toward the ceiling to stretch your abdominal muscles.

Make it easier: Lift without rotating.
Make it harder: Lift your toes up, keeping your heels on the floor, as you do the exercise.

STABILITY BALL WORKOUT

3 Arm V-lift on stability ball

Reps: 10
Sets: 1–3
Tempo: 3-1-3
Rest: 30–90 seconds between sets

Starting position: Lie on your stomach on a stability ball with your hands on the floor in front of you and your legs extended behind you, feet hip-width apart. Keep the ball centered under your waist.

Movement: Exhale as you lift your hands toward the ceiling, thumbs pointing up, until your body is in a straight line from the top of your head to your heels. Hold. Return to the starting position.

Tips and techniques:
- Keep your neck neutral throughout the movement.
- Keep your spine neutral; don't arch it.
- Tighten your shoulder blades as you lift your arms up.

Make it easier: Lift one arm at a time.
Make it harder: Do an additional 10 lifts with your arms extended out to the sides.

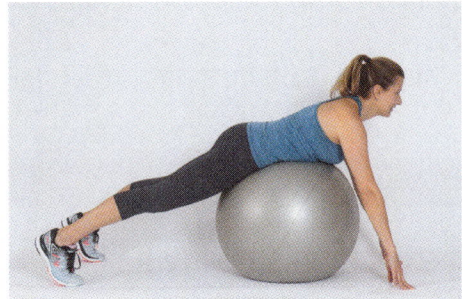
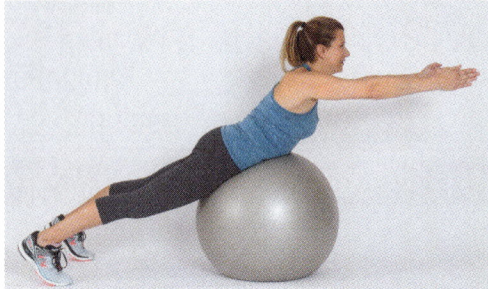

4 Knee tuck on stability ball

Reps: 10
Sets: 1–3
Tempo: 3-1-3
Rest: 30–90 seconds between sets

Starting position: Lie on your stomach on a stability ball with your hands on the floor in front of you. Walk your hands out until you are in a comfortable plank position with your shins on the ball and your hands directly under your shoulders.

Movement: Contracting your abdominal muscles, bend your knees and pull them and the ball in toward your chest. Hold. Straighten your legs to return to the starting position.

Tips and techniques:
- Keep your head and spine neutral.
- Keep your shoulders down and back, away from your ears.

For a demonstration of this exercise, go to www.health.harvard.edu/knee-tuck.

Make it easier: Don't pull your knees in as far.
Make it harder: Hold the tucked position for a count of three before returning to the starting position.

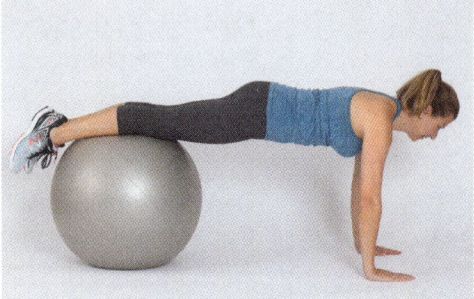
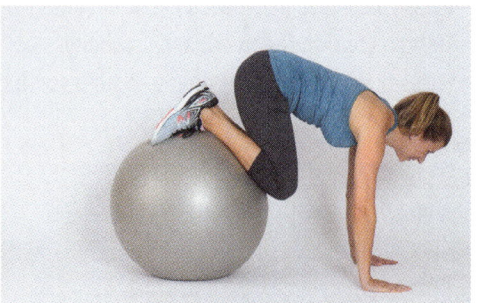

36 Core Exercises www.health.harvard.edu

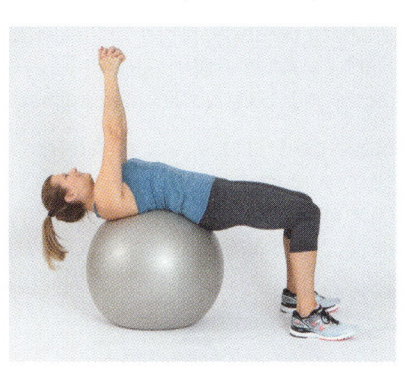

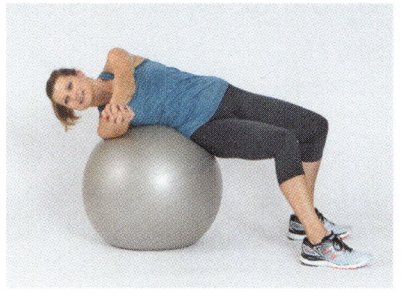

STABILITY BALL WORKOUT

5 Front plank on stability ball

Reps: 2–4
Sets: 1
Hold: 15–60 seconds
Rest: 30–90 seconds between reps

Starting position: Kneel on the floor. Place your forearms on top of the stability ball, elbows bent.

Movement: Tighten your abdominal muscles as you lift your knees off the floor and extend your body into a plank position with your legs straight and the balls of your feet on the floor. Hold.

Tips and techniques:
- Keep your shoulders aligned with your elbows.
- Keep your neck and spine neutral.
- Keep your shoulders down and back to stabilize your shoulder blades.

Make it easier: Perform the plank with your knees on the floor, with your body in a straight line from head to knees.
Make it harder: Move the ball slightly forward and back, side to side, or in circles while performing the plank.

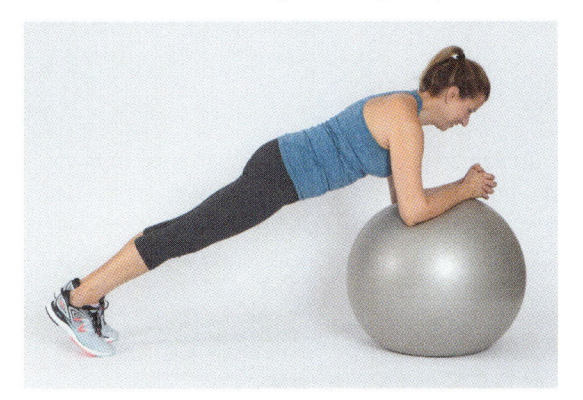

6 Torso rotation on stability ball

Reps: 10
Sets: 1–3
Tempo: 3–1–3
Rest: 30–90 seconds between sets

Starting position: Sit on the stability ball. Lean back and roll downward, walking your feet forward until the ball is centered under your back. Position your feet shoulder-width apart with your knees aligned directly over your ankles. Clasp your hands together and extend your arms toward the ceiling above your chest.

Movement: Keeping your arms extended, rotate your head, arms, and torso to the right. Hold. Return to the starting position. Repeat, rotating to the left. That completes one rep.

Tips and techniques:
- Engage your core by squeezing your buttocks and tightening your abdominal muscles.
- As you rotate your torso, your upper shoulder will come off the ball.
- Keep your feet still throughout the movement.

Make it easier: Rotate less, or lower just one arm to the side, allowing your head to follow.
Make it harder: Roll farther off the ball so only your head and upper back are supported. Or, hold a medicine ball or dumbbell as you perform the exercise.

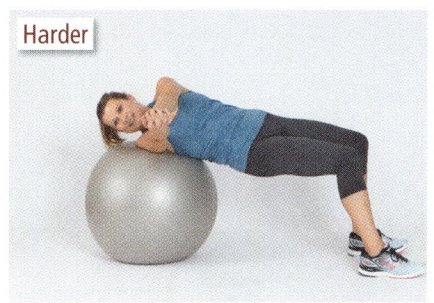

Harder

www.health.harvard.edu Core Exercises 37

STABILITY BALL WORKOUT

7 Deadbug with stability ball

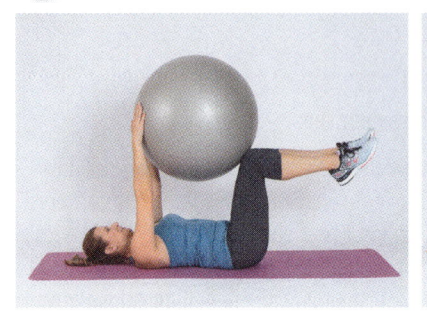

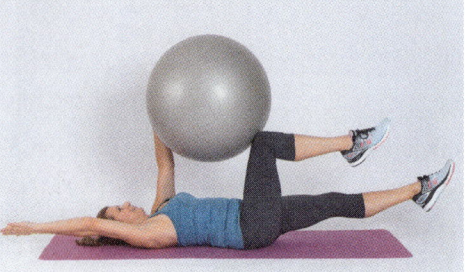

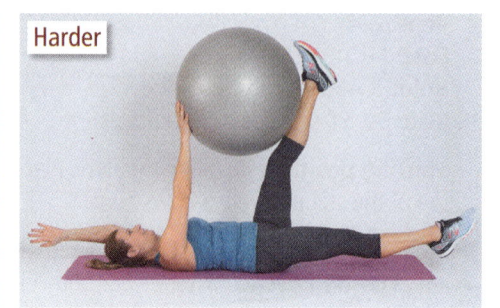

Reps: 10
Sets: 1–3
Tempo: 3-1-3
Rest: 30–90 seconds between sets

Starting position: Lie on your back with your feet off the floor and hips and knees bent at 90°. Take the stability ball and place it over your body, holding it in place with your hands and knees.

Movement: Extend your left leg and right arm down toward the floor so you're balancing the ball with your left hand and right knee only. Hold. Return to the starting position and repeat with the opposite arm and leg. That's one rep.

Tips and techniques:
- Keep your spine neutral and your shoulders down and back.
- Engage your core by contracting your abdominal muscles.
- Keep your head on the mat.

Make it easier: Make the movements small, not lowering your arm and leg so close to the floor.
Make it harder: Do the exercise with your legs extended straight up to the ceiling, holding the stability ball between your lower legs and hands.

8 Bridge extensions and curls

Reps: 10
Sets: 1–3
Tempo: 3-1-3
Rest: 30–90 seconds between sets

Starting position: Lie on your back on the floor with your knees bent, feet flat on the upper side of a stability ball, and your arms down at your sides. Shift into the bridge position by tightening your buttocks and pressing your feet into the stability ball to lift your hips, lower back, and middle back off the floor.

Movement: Straighten your legs to roll the ball away from you while keeping your core still and stable. Hold. Then pull the ball back toward you by bending your knees and pressing your heels into the ball. Complete all reps before lowering your hips back to the floor.

Tips and techniques:
- Keep your spine neutral and avoid arching your back.
- Avoid locking your knees as you extend your legs on the ball.
- Keep your hips even.

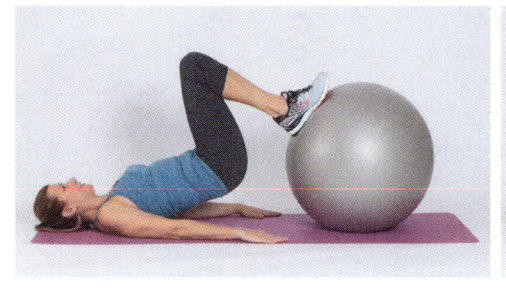

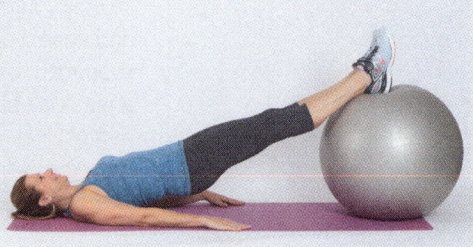

Make it easier: Lower your hips to the floor between reps, as needed.
Make it harder: Do the moves with your arms crossed on your chest.

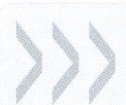

>>> **You're not done yet** See "Finish with stretches," page 43, for a set of seven stretches to end your routine. Stretching helps to prevent stiffness and preserve flexibility and range of motion.

38 Core Exercises www.health.harvard.edu

Bosu Workout

Ready for a new challenge after mastering the Stability Ball Workout? The curved dome of the Bosu forces muscles from your ankles up through your shoulders and neck to work in concert so you can hold a position steadily and move smoothly through each core exercise. This workout improves your balance, which pays off when reaching and rotating in sports like tennis and golf or when walking and running on uneven terrain. But you should do this workout only if you already have very good balance. Exercising on the Bosu is much more challenging than the previous workouts and has more potential for falls, if you are not able to fine-tune your balance from moment to moment.

Focus on good form. If you find an exercise especially difficult, do fewer reps or try the easier variation. For a more vigorous workout, try the harder variation. Remember to begin with a short warm-up (see "Warm up," page 9).

Equipment: Bosu Balance Trainer; mat or carpet for comfort (last exercise only).

BOSU WORKOUT

1 Bosu squat

Reps: 10
Sets: 1–3
Tempo: 3–1–3
Rest: 30–90 seconds between sets

Starting position: Stand up straight on top of the Bosu with your feet hip-width apart, arms at your sides. Try to stand evenly on both feet, pressing your big toes into the Bosu.

Movement: Hinge forward at your hips and bend your knees to lower your buttocks as if sitting down in a chair. Simultaneously, bring your hands forward in front of your chest. Stop with your buttocks above knee level. Hold. Return to the starting position.

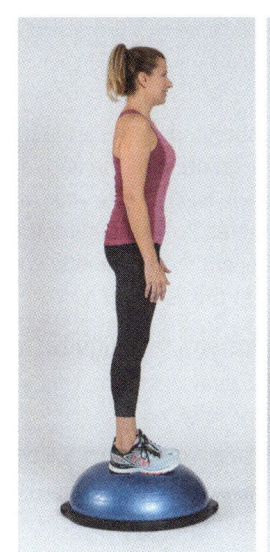

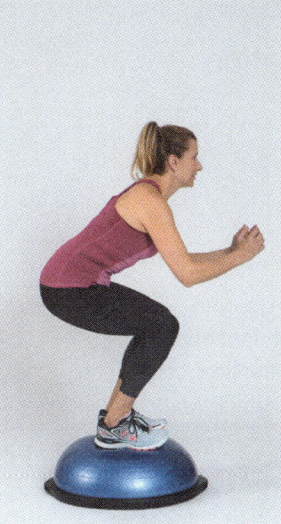

Tips and techniques:
- Keep your hips, knees, and toes pointing forward and your spine neutral.
- Your knees should extend no farther than your toes.
- Keep your chest lifted and your shoulders down and back.

Make it easier: Make the squat smaller, lowering only halfway.
Make it harder: Hold the squat for four counts.

www.health.harvard.edu   Core Exercises   39

BOSU WORKOUT

2 Alternating knee lifts

Reps: 10
Sets: 1–3
Tempo: 3–1–3
Rest: 30–90 seconds between sets

Starting position: Stand up straight on top of the Bosu with your feet together and arms extended out to your sides at shoulder height.

Movement: Tighten your abdominal muscles and buttocks for stability. Lift your left knee up toward the ceiling as high as is comfortable with good posture. Hold. Then lower it to the starting position. Repeat with the right knee. This is one rep.

Tips and techniques:
- Keep your chest lifted and your shoulders down and back.
- Gaze at a stationary spot in front of you to help with balance. If you lose your balance, take a moment to stabilize yourself and then continue.
- Keep your pelvis stable as you lift your knee. If you notice any shifting, don't lift as high.

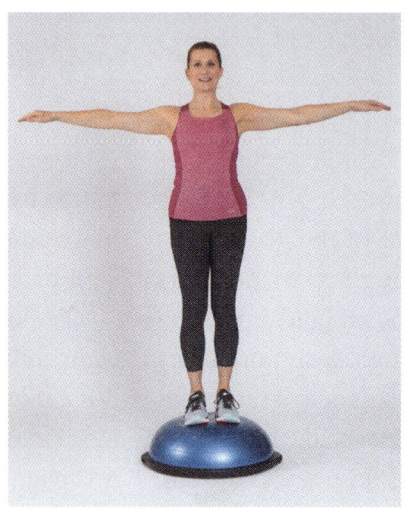

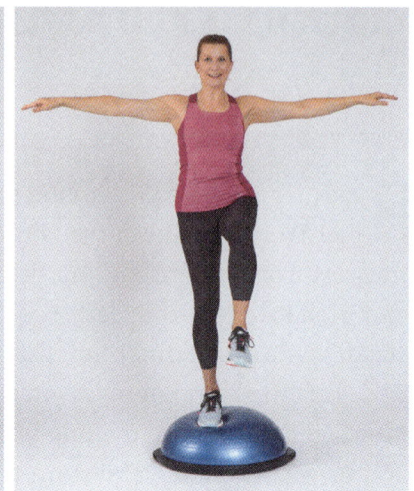

Make it easier: Don't lift each knee as high.
Make it harder: Hold each knee lift for four counts.

3 Reverse lunge with rotation

Reps: 10
Sets: 1–3
Tempo: 2–2–2–2
Rest: 30–90 seconds between sets

Starting position: Stand up straight with feet together on top of the Bosu, arms at your sides.

Movement: Step backward with your left foot off the Bosu, placing the ball of your foot and toes on the floor behind you. Bend your knees and sink into a lunge position, while bringing your hands together in front of your chest. Your left knee should be pointing to the floor and your right thigh about parallel to the floor. Next, rotate your torso to the right, and then come back to center. Push off your left foot to return to the starting position. Repeat the lunge with your right leg, rotating your torso to the left. This is one rep.

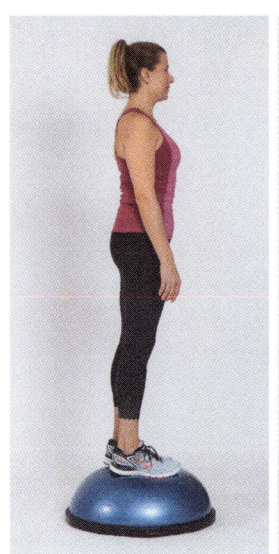

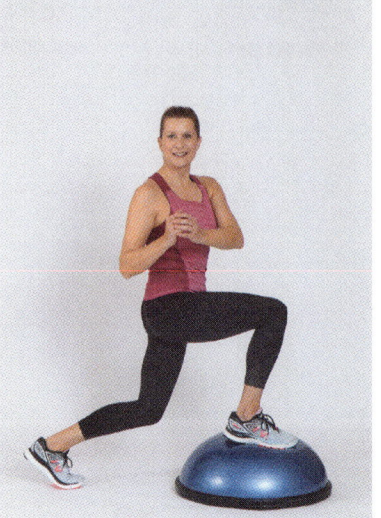

Tips and techniques:
- Evenly distribute your weight over both feet in the lunge position.
- Keep your front knee behind your toes.
- Keep your chest lifted, shoulders back and down, and spine neutral.
- Tighten your abdominal muscles and buttocks for stability.

Make it easier: Skip the torso rotation.
Make it harder: Hold the torso rotation for four counts.

BOSU WORKOUT

4 Diagonal opposite arm and leg raise

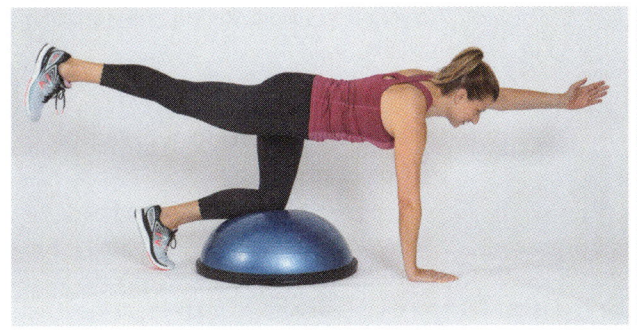

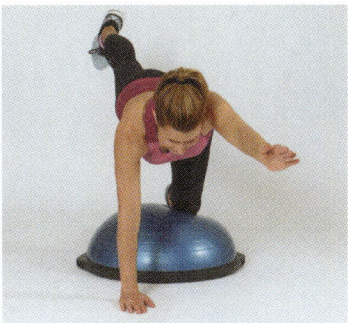

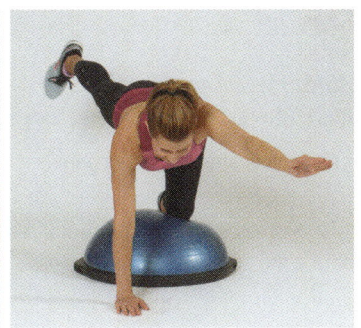

Reps: 10
Sets: 1–3
Tempo: 2–4–2
Rest: 30–90 seconds between sets

Starting position: Kneel with your knees on the Bosu and directly under your hips, toes resting on the floor behind you. Place both hands on the floor in front of you, directly under your shoulders.

Movement: Extend your right leg off the floor behind you as you simultaneously reach out in front of you with your left arm, thumb up. Keeping your shoulders and hips squared, move your left arm to the left and your right leg to the right for a greater balance challenge. (If you imagine a clock with your head being 12, your left arm would be at about 10 and your right leg at about 4.) Hold for a count of four. Then, bring your arm and leg back in and slowly lower them to the starting position. Repeat with your right arm (2 o'clock position) and left leg (8 o'clock position). This is one rep.

Tips and techniques:
- As you lift, think of creating a straight line from your fingers to your toes.
- Keep your neck and spine neutral.
- Tighten your abdominal muscles for stability.

For a demonstration of this exercise, go to www.health.harvard.edu/diagonal-raise.

Make it easier: Lift your arm straight in front of you and your leg straight behind you. Don't move them out to the sides.
Make it harder: Lift the toes of the leg resting on the Bosu off the floor.

5 Side squat with leg lift

Reps: 10 per side
Sets: 1–3
Tempo: 3–1–3
Rest: 30–90 seconds between sets

Starting position: Stand up straight with your arms at your sides, your right foot on top of the Bosu, and your left foot on the floor, feet about hip-width apart. Center your body weight between your feet.

Movement: Hinge forward at your hips and bend your knees to lower your buttocks as if sitting down in a chair, stopping with your buttocks above knee level. Simultaneously, bring your hands together in front of your chest. Hold. As you straighten your legs, shift your weight onto the right leg (the one on the Bosu), and lift your left leg and both arms out to the sides. Lower your left leg and arms, returning to the squat position. This is one rep. Finish all reps, then repeat with your left foot on the Bosu. That's one set.

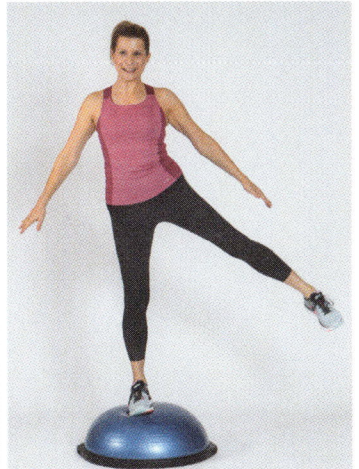

Tips and techniques:
- Keep your spine neutral and your shoulders down and back.
- Keep your hips and the knees and toes of the supporting leg pointing forward.
- Tighten the buttock of the leg on top of the Bosu for stability as you lift up and extend the other leg.

Make it easier: Make the movements smaller.
Make it harder: Hold the leg lift for two counts.

www.health.harvard.edu Core Exercises 41

BOSU WORKOUT

6 Front plank on Bosu

Reps: 2–4
Sets: 1
Hold: 15–60 seconds
Rest: 30–90 seconds between reps

Starting position: Place your forearms on top of the Bosu with your elbows under your shoulders, hands loosely clasped, and knees on the floor with your toes tucked under.

Movement: Tighten your abdominal muscles as you lift your knees off the floor and extend your lower body into a full plank position. Your body should be in line from the top of your head to your heels. Hold. Return to the starting position.

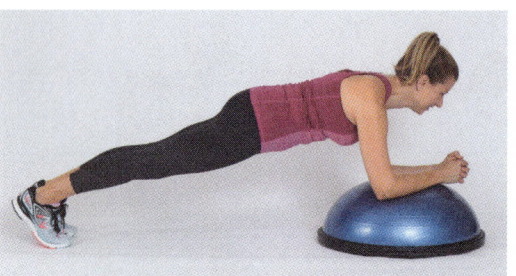

Tips and techniques:
- Keep your head and spine neutral.
- Don't bend at your hips.
- Keep your shoulders down and back, over your elbows.

Make it easier: Perform the plank with your knees on the floor. Be sure your body is in line from head to knees.
Make it harder: While holding the plank position, lift one leg for four counts, then the other leg for four counts. Continue repeating this throughout the plank.

7 Single-leg bridge

Reps: 10 per side
Sets: 1–3
Tempo: 3–1–3
Rest: 30–90 seconds between sets

Starting position: Lie on your back with your knees bent. Place your right foot on top of the Bosu and extend your left foot straight up toward the ceiling. Rest your arms at your sides on the floor.

Movement: Tighten your buttocks as you lift your hips off the floor. Hold. Lower your buttocks to the floor. Complete all reps with this leg extended, then repeat with the left foot on the Bosu and your right leg extended. That's one set.

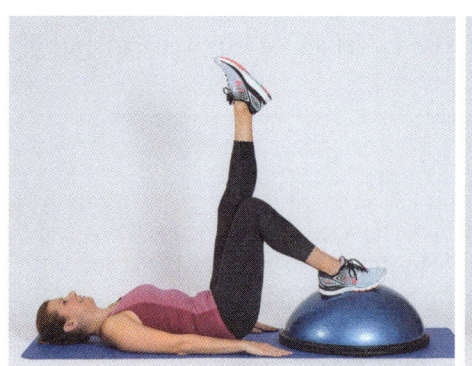

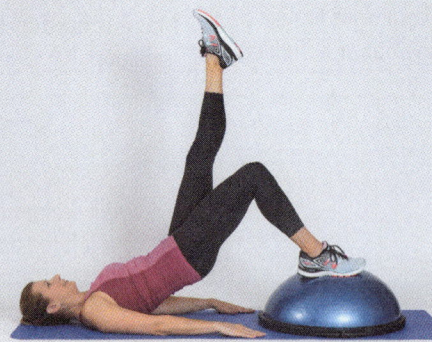

Tips and techniques:
- Keep your spine neutral.
- Keep your shoulders, hips, and knees in line in the bridge.
- Don't lift too high; keep your upper back on the floor.

Make it easier: Perform a bridge with both feet on the Bosu.
Make it harder: Hold each single-leg bridge for four counts.

>>> **You're not done yet** See "Finish with stretches," page 43, for a set of seven stretches to end your routine. Stretching helps to prevent stiffness and preserve flexibility and range of motion.

Finish with stretches

You're not done until you've stretched. It takes only a few moves to stay limber. End your workouts by doing these seven stretches to increase your range of motion and to relax after a good workout.

To perform the stretches: Be sure to hold each stretch for 10 to 30 seconds and repeat it three or four times. If you hold the position for less time or do fewer repetitions, you won't lengthen the muscle fibers as effectively. On the other hand, holding a stretch for too long can increase your chances of injuring the muscle. When you are starting out, you may find that it's useful to time your stretches.

Here are some other safety tips:
- While stretching, remember to breathe normally (unless instructed otherwise).
- Don't bounce.
- Don't lock your knees or elbows.
- Don't overextend your body. Stretch only to the point of mild tension, never pain. If a stretch hurts, stop immediately.
- Stretches should be felt in the middle of a muscle, not in the joints.

Equipment: Yoga strap or belt; chair; mat or carpet for comfort.

STRETCHES

1 Quadriceps stretch

Reps: 3–4
Sets: 1
Hold: 10–30 seconds

Starting position: Stand up straight with your feet together. Place your right hand on the back of a chair.

Movement: Bend your left knee and bring the heel of your left foot toward your left buttock. Grasp your left foot with your left hand. (If that's not possible, loop a strap or belt around your foot and hold on to that.) Hold. Slowly lower your foot to the floor. Repeat with your right leg. This is one rep.

Where you'll feel it: Front of thigh

Tips and techniques:
- Your bent knee should point directly down toward the floor, not out to the side.
- Don't arch your back.

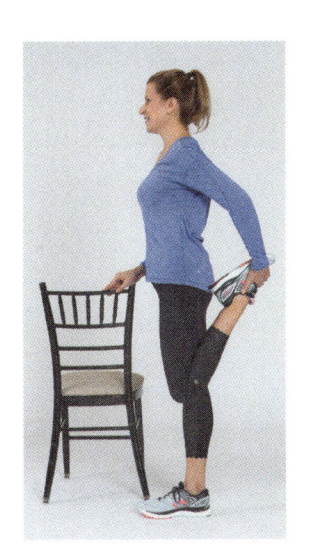

2 Chest stretch

Reps: 3–4
Sets: 1
Hold: 10–30 seconds

Starting position: Stand up straight with your feet about hip-width apart. Clasp your hands together behind your back.

Movement: Lift your hands up and away from your body, until you feel the stretch. Hold. Return to the starting position.

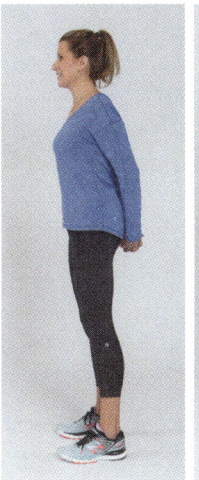

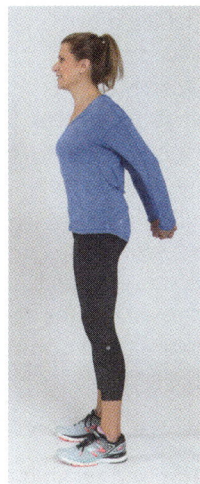

Where you'll feel it: Chest and shoulders

Tips and techniques:
- Keep your shoulders down and back.
- Don't lean forward as you lift.
- Don't arch your back; maintain a neutral spine.

STRETCHES

3 Hamstring stretch

Reps: 3–4
Sets: 1
Hold: 10–30 seconds

Starting position: Lie on your back with your left knee bent and your left foot on the floor. Loop a strap or belt around your right foot.

Movement: Flex your right foot and extend your leg toward the ceiling. Pull on the strap until you feel a stretch. Hold. Return to the starting position and repeat with the left leg. This is one rep.

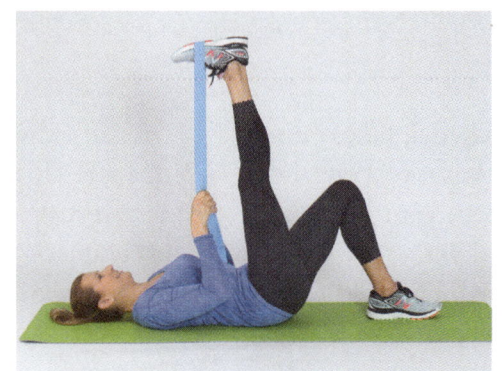

Where you'll feel it: Back of thigh

Tips and techniques:
- Straighten your leg as much as possible without locking the knee.
- You can straighten the leg that's on the floor for a deeper stretch.

4 Torso rotation stretch

Reps: 3–4
Sets: 1
Hold: 10–30 seconds

Starting position: Lie on your back with your knees bent and your feet together flat on the floor. Extend your arms comfortably out to each side just below shoulder level.

Movement: Tighten your abdominal muscles as you lower both knees together toward the floor on the left side. Keeping your shoulders relaxed and pressed into the floor, turn your head to the right. Hold. Return to the starting position. Repeat in the opposite direction. This is one rep.

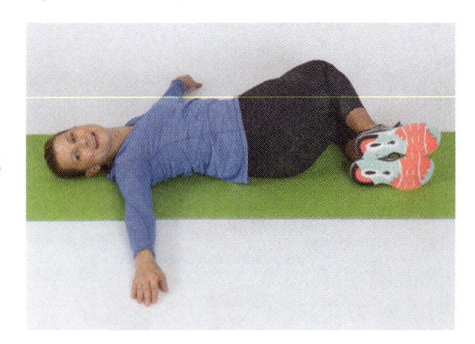

Where you'll feel it: Chest and torso

Tips and techniques:
- If your knees don't comfortably rest on the floor, place a pillow or folded blanket under them.
- Keep your shoulders down on the floor.

5 Hip stretch

Reps: 3–4
Sets: 1
Hold: 10–30 seconds

Starting position: Lie on your back with your left knee bent and your left foot on the floor. Rest your right ankle on your left thigh, close to the kneecap. Your right knee should point out to the side.

Movement: Grasp the back of your left thigh with both hands and lift your left foot off the floor until you feel a stretch in your right outer hip and buttock. Hold. Return to the starting position. Repeat on the other side. This is one rep.

Where you'll feel it: Outside of hip and buttocks

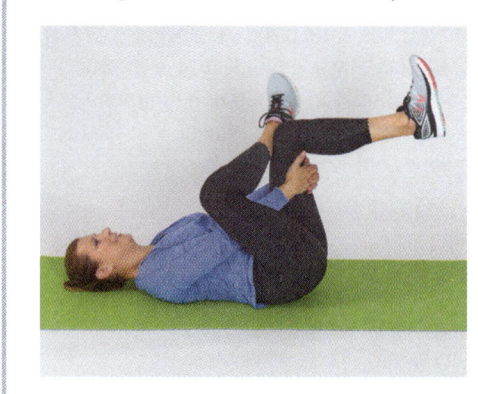

Tips and techniques:
- Keep your shoulders back and down, away from your ears.
- Keep your head on the floor.

STRETCHES

6 Cat-cow

Reps: 8–10
Sets: 1
Tempo: 4–4

Starting position: Get down on all fours, with your hands directly beneath your shoulders and your knees beneath your hips. Keep your spine neutral.

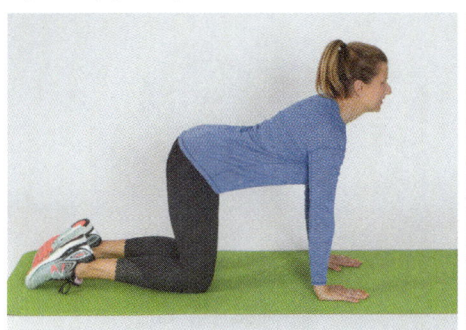

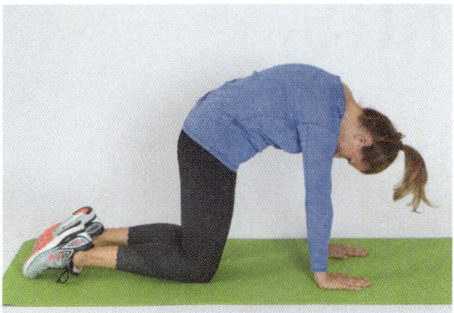

Movement: Inhale and lift your chest and tailbone toward the ceiling like a cow. As you exhale, round your back, bringing your chin toward your chest and tucking your tailbone under like a cat. That's one rep. Continue moving with your breath; do not hold.

Where you'll feel it: Chest, back, hamstrings

Tips and techniques:
- Keep the movement slow and controlled.
- Don't overarch your back.
- If you have back problems or osteoporosis, check with your doctor before doing this move.

7 Child's pose stretch with diagonal reach

Reps: 3–4
Sets: 1
Hold: 10–30 seconds

Starting position: Kneel on all fours, knees hip-width apart, big toes touching, and head and neck in neutral alignment.

Movement: This is a three-part stretch. (1) Slowly lower your buttocks back toward your heels as you extend your hands in front of you and rest your forehead on the mat. Hold. (2) Walk your hands out to the left so your upper body is on a diagonal, and place your right hand on top of your left hand. Hold. (3) Walk your hands out to the right and place your left hand on top of your right hand. Hold. Walk your hands back to the center and return to the starting position. That's one rep.

Where you'll feel it: Back, shoulders, and sides of torso

Tips and techniques:
- Keep your head down, so you are looking at the floor.
- Place a pillow or a rolled towel between your thighs and calves if you can't sit back all the way.
- Breathe comfortably.

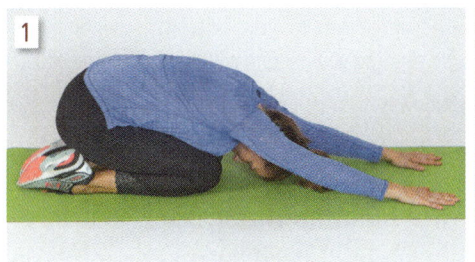

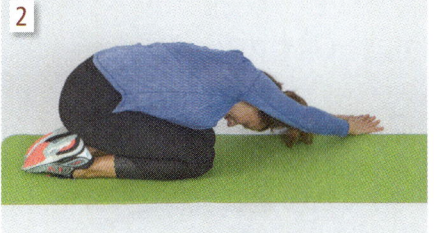

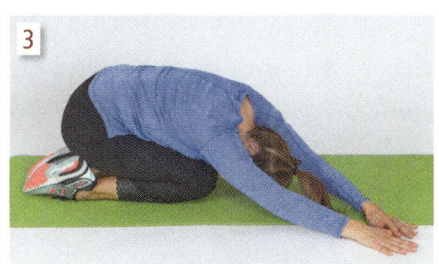

SPECIAL SECTION

Setting goals, motivating yourself, and maintaining gains

Maybe you're the kind of person who can just dive right in to a new workout and maintain your motivation to keep it up. But for many people, setting formal goals and finding tricks to help stay on track will make the difference between success and failure. This chapter is your guide to success. It will help you set smart goals, carve out time to exercise, and rev up motivation. Exercising consistently is sometimes hard, so we've highlighted tips to help you identify—and smooth out—likely bumps in the road.

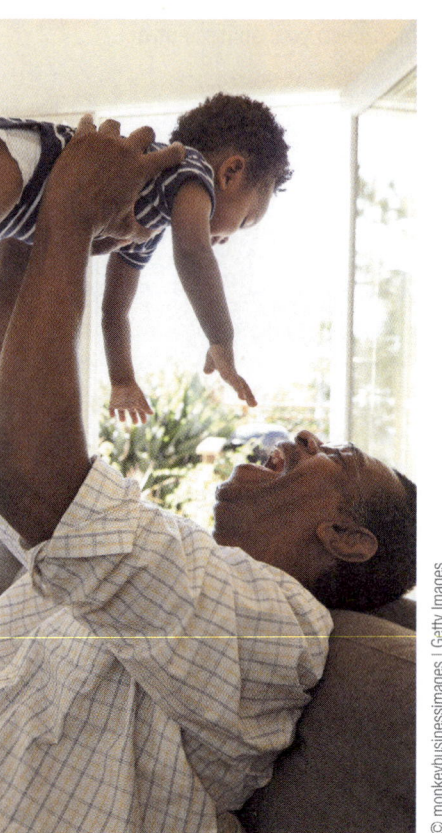

Having a goal can help keep you motivated to do core work. The goal might be anything from improving your posture to building the strength you need to play with the grandkids..

When you're ready to pick up the challenge a little, you'll find tips at the end of the chapter on how to progress to the next level and how to maintain your gains.

Choose a goal

How will adding core work to your activities benefit you? Check off your goals from the options in the following list, and write a personalized goal in the space provided in "Make your commitment" on page 49. For example, *I want to*

❏ keep my back strong and flexible in order to help me avoid lower back pain
❏ ease back pain or stiffness so I can move, sit, and sleep comfortably
❏ reclaim the strength and flexibility I need for everyday tasks like bending, turning, lifting, yanking, reaching items on high shelves, and the many actions required for gardening, fix-it work, and housework
❏ build up the strength and flexibility I need for on-the-job tasks like lifting heavy items, twisting, or standing or sitting at a desk for hours
❏ add power for athletic activities I enjoy like tennis or other racquet sports, a marathon or triathlon, golf, kayaking, and other active pursuits

46   Core Exercises

www.health.harvard.edu

Setting goals, motivating yourself, and maintaining gains | **SPECIAL SECTION**

- enhance my balance and stability, which will help prevent falls
- improve my posture, which can trim my figure visually, make clothes fit well, ease the stress of desk and computer work, and help prevent back injuries
- help tone my waistline (when combined with diet and other measures; see "Your waistline: A measure of health," page 5)
- buff my muscles for six-pack abs (see "Building a better six-pack," page 15)
- spice up my weekly workouts by adding variation.

Be SMART

As you know by now, fitting core exercises into your life will pay off in everyday activities, sports successes, a stronger lower back, independent living, and all-around fitness. Even so, if you're not in the habit of working out, it may not be easy for you to marshal the time and will to do these exercises on a regular basis. Experts say you're more likely to meet success if you set goals that are SMART—that is, specific, measurable, achievable, realistic, and time-based. So as you're setting a goal and penciling it in on the calendar we've provided, make sure it passes the SMART test, described below.

S Set a very **specific** goal—for example, *I will do the Standing Core Workout on Monday and Wednesday.* Or, *I will do a set of front and side planks on Tuesday, Thursday, and Sunday.*

M Find a way to **measure** your success—for instance, *I will log my efforts daily on my calendar, checking off days when I met my goal* (see "My monthly activity calendar," page 50).

A Make sure it's **achievable**. Are you physically capable of safely accomplishing your goal? If not, aim for a smaller goal initially. Instead of starting off with the Bosu Workout, for example, start with the Floor Core and Standing Core workouts, which are easier since the exercises are done on a stable surface.

R Make sure it's **realistic**. On a scale of 1 to 10, where 1 equals no confidence in your ability to meet your goal and 10 equals 100% certainty, your goal should land in the 7–10 zone. If it's not in that range, cut it down to a manageable size. For example, *I'll add five minutes of core exercises to my regular strength routine* might be more realistic for you than aiming for 20 minutes of core three days a week on top of everything else.

T Set **time** commitments. Pick a date and time to start—for example, *Starting this week, I'll get up half an hour earlier on Wednesday and Friday to do the Floor Core Workout.* Also choose a weekly check-in time to keep track of whether you're meeting goals or hitting snags: *I'll check my calendar every Friday evening and decide if I should make any changes in my routines to succeed.* Outside deadlines can be really helpful here, too: signing up for a tennis tournament or knowing you'll need to wiggle into beach clothes in six weeks prods you to get your core program under way.

Motivate yourself

Usually, we do our best work when motivated. That extends to exercise, too. It's not uncommon to launch a new exercise program raring to go, only to wind up back on the couch with your feet propped up just a few weeks later. If your will wavers, the tips here may help.

Refresh your memory. Remind yourself how the exercises will help you by reading your goals again. Emphasize the positive aspects. Rather than sternly saying, "I should do my core workout," try saying aloud "My back feels better when I do my core exercises," or "My backhand and serve are much stronger when I do my core exercises consistently."

Find the time. Skimming time from your busy schedule is an art. Here are some ideas for carving out the time for a full workout:

- Over the course of a week, skip two half-hour TV shows, or exercise while you watch.
- Get up half an hour earlier each day to do a full workout.
- Be efficient: a short, challenging workout tunes up core muscles just as well, if not better, than racking up set after set of easier exercises. As you advance to more challenging exercises,

www.health.harvard.edu

Core Exercises

SPECIAL SECTION | Setting goals, motivating yourself, and maintaining gains

leave the simpler ones behind to make the best use of your time.

Slip core activities into your day. Throughout the day, be on the lookout for pockets of time. While on the phone, do side leg lifts or pliés. Before shifting from calls to other projects or back again, do a few front or side planks. Spend the first five minutes of your lunch break doing leg swings, reverse lunges, squats with knee lifts. For more ideas, see "Finding the time" on page 13.

Plan simple rewards. Give yourself a pat on the back for every small or big step toward success. Blast your favorite tune at the end of a workout. Text a friend after a workout so he or she can cheer you on. Treat yourself to a relaxing bath before bed with a beautifully scented bath oil. A bigger reward for staying on track toward your goal for two to four weeks might be new workout gear or sports equipment or a massage.

Get a workout buddy. Workouts with a friend or family member are more fun, plus you're less likely to cancel on the spur of the moment. Or, if you belong to a gym, ask if there is a buddy program. At home, you could arrange to do core workouts with a distant friend via Skype.

If finding a real-time or virtual workout buddy isn't possible, do the next best thing: find a core-focused exercise class at the gym (look for class names like Core Focus or Hard Core). Working out with others can be fun, and the connections you make will keep you coming back.

Reach for your smartphone or iPad. Yet another option is a livestream or on-demand workout through Forte, Daily Burn, or iFit. Most require a subscription, but Nike Training Club offers free workouts. Another option is to try a fitness game on an older system like Wii or Xbox or a newer virtual reality system like Oculus or PlayStation VR. Some of the activities they offer—like tennis, dancing, and dodging obstacles—will work your core. You can find fitness games at local gaming shops, large

Overcoming obstacles

Brainstorming solutions for likely bumps in the road can start you off on the right foot and help keep workouts on track. Once you get going, jot down any hurdles you run into on your monthly activity calendar and then think your way around them. Here's some help with common problems.

Need the okay to start doing core exercises? Call your doctor today. It may help to fax or email a copy of the workouts you hope to do, then follow up with a phone call to discuss whether any modifications will be needed.

Don't belong to a gym (or can't seem to get to one)? Try the Standing Core Workout, Floor Core Workout, or Pilates Workout, which require no equipment. Or buy the equipment necessary for doing certain core workouts at home. Start with the less expensive items, such as a medicine ball or a stability ball.

Just don't feel motivated? Ask a friend to check up on you or have a friendly competition with you. Working out with a personal trainer is another option.

Bored by your routine? If you've mastered the basic moves, try the harder variations. Or change over to another workout entirely. Tried them all? Mix and match one or two moves from each workout to create a completely new routine.

Not yet buff enough to make it through a workout? Try one or more of these options:

- Focus on the easy variations of exercises you find too hard.
- Start with fewer reps (or holding a position like a plank for fewer seconds). When that becomes easy, do additional reps or hold longer.
- Start with Short Workout 1 or Short Workout 2 (see "Four short workouts," page 13).
- Do just half of the exercises in a workout twice a week. Each week, try to add another exercise until you're doing the full workout.

Still stuck? Sometimes breaking a bigger goal down is the best way to succeed. For example, instead of trying for two complete core workouts per week, use the options in the previous tip to break down a big workout into more manageable steps.

Core Exercises   www.health.harvard.edu

Setting goals, motivating yourself, and maintaining gains | **SPECIAL SECTION**

retailers, and online stores. For your smartphone, look for fitness app options at Apple's App Store or Google Play. On the Web, try the American Council on Exercise fitness library (www.acefitness.org/exerciselibrary) or other virtual trainer and interactive tools.

Make your commitment

Now, put your SMART goal and plans together into a commitment statement. Here's an example:

I'm making a commitment to my health, well-being, and enjoyment of life. My goal is to improve my balance. I plan to start on Tuesday, May 15, by doing the Standing Core Workout. I will do it every Tuesday and Friday at 6:30 a.m. I'll check my activity calendar weekly on Sunday nights to see if I'm succeeding. If not, I'll brainstorm ways to overcome obstacles and motivate myself to get back on track.

Now you try

I'm making a commitment to my health, well-being, and enjoyment of life. My goal is _____
_____.

I plan to start on _____
by doing _____
on _____.

I'll check my activity calendar weekly on _____ to see if I'm succeeding. If not, I'll brainstorm ways to overcome obstacles and motivate myself to get back on track.

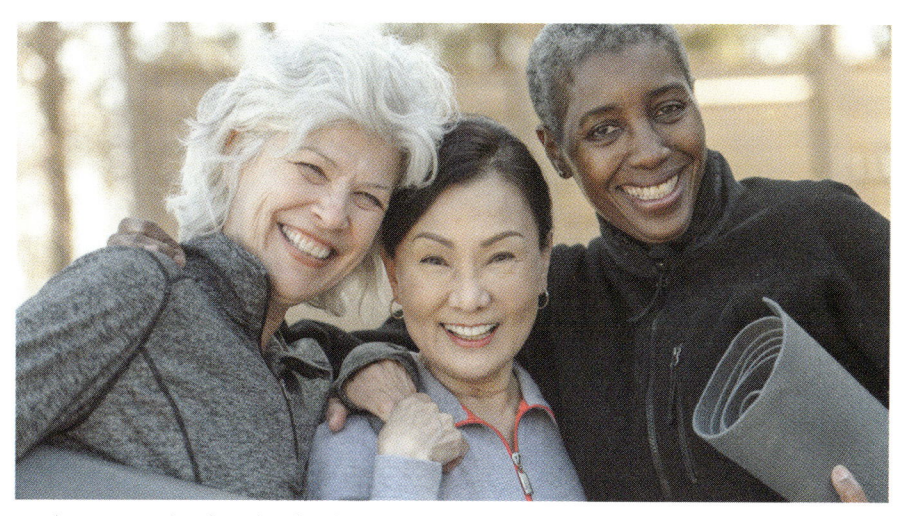

Working out with a friend or family member is more fun than working out alone—plus you're less likely to skip a session if you know that someone else is counting on you to be there. Other options include gym classes or even working out with a buddy via Skype.

Take it up a notch

As you repeat a core workout over time, you will notice that the exercises become easier to do. At a certain point, you will want to increase the level of difficulty, so that you continue to make gains. But how do you know when you're ready to move on? You're ready to progress if you can manage all four of these tasks throughout each exercise:

- maintain good form
- stick to the specified tempo
- use a full, or comfortable, range of motion
- complete the suggested number of reps or hold the position for the suggested number of seconds.

At that point, you can step up the challenge of any given workout by making one of these choices:

- adding sets (up to three)
- adding resistance (such as a heavier medicine ball)
- trying the harder variation of the exercise (see the "Make it harder" options in the workouts).

Maintain your gains

At some point, you may be satisfied with the gains you've made. To maintain those gains, stick to the highest level of challenge you've achieved and do a core workout at least once a week. Or, if you usually do bursts of core work throughout the day, continue that routine.

If you get sick or take time off for other reasons, you may need to drop down a level—that is, choose less resistance or do fewer reps and sets—and then build up again.

What if your routine no longer feels challenging? That's a signal that you need to step it up again if you want to maintain gains you've made. And if you begin to feel bored, go over your goals again. Then vary your core work by trying a new workout or selecting new exercises to do throughout the day.

www.health.harvard.edu

Core Exercises

My monthly activity calendar

Make copies of the blank calendar below so that you'll be able to fill it out each month. Put each month's calendar in an easy-to-see spot. Then follow these instructions:

Month _____

1. Use the notes space to the right to jot down your commitment and your rewards.

2. Pencil in days and times you plan to do core work, and what you'll be doing (for example, bursts of exercise or a particular workout). Remember, core work should be part of a larger exercise plan, as explained in "How does core work fit into your exercise plans?" on page 12. So, when penciling in your core exercise schedule, it makes sense to write down other

SUNDAY	MONDAY	TUESDAY	WEDNESDAY

strength sessions and aerobic activities, too.

3. Put a big splashy check mark next to each success. Anytime you fall short, record the obstacle in the notes section, then try to brainstorm and jot down a solution (see "Overcoming obstacles," page 48).

4. Once a week, look over what you've checked off. Think about what's working well for you. Decide whether your solutions for overcoming hurdles are working, or whether you need to break your goal down into smaller steps in order to be successful (see "Overcoming obstacles," page 48). And collect any reward due, as planned.

THURSDAY	FRIDAY	SATURDAY

MY COMMITMENT

OBSTACLES

SOLUTIONS

REWARDS

Resources

Organizations

American Academy of Physical Medicine and Rehabilitation
9700 W. Bryn Mawr Ave., Suite 200
Rosemont, IL 60018
847-737-6000
www.aapmr.org

This professional organization for physiatrists (medical doctors trained in physical medicine and rehabilitation) provides information on conditions such as low back and neck pain and osteoporosis. A referral service on the website can help you locate physiatrists near you.

American College of Sports Medicine
401 W. Michigan St.
Indianapolis, IN 46202
317-637-9200
www.acsm.org

ACSM is a nonprofit that educates and certifies fitness professionals, such as personal trainers, and offers information to the public on various types of exercise. A referral service on the website lists ACSM-certified personal trainers (click on "Get & Stay Certified," then "Find a Pro").

American Council on Exercise
4851 Paramount Drive
San Diego, CA 92123
888-825-3636 (toll-free)
www.acefitness.org

ACE is a nonprofit organization that promotes fitness and offers a wide array of educational materials for consumers and professionals. The website has a referral service to help locate ACE-certified personal trainers and health coaches and a library of free exercise videos.

American Physical Therapy Association
1111 N. Fairfax St.
Alexandria, VA 22314
800-999-2782 (toll-free)
www.apta.org

This national professional organization fosters advances in education, research, and the practice of physical therapy. The website has a search engine to help locate board-certified clinical specialists who have additional training in specific areas of physical therapy.

Harvard Special Health Reports

If you're looking for more exercises, the following reports from Harvard Medical School can help. They can be ordered online at www.health.harvard.edu or by calling 877–649–9457 (toll-free).

Better Balance: Simple exercises to improve stability and prevent falls
Suzanne Salamon, M.D., and Brad Manor, Ph.D., Medical Editors
(Harvard Medical School, 2017)

This report provides six complete workouts to improve balance, starting with three easy balance workouts and progressing through three harder workouts. Two workouts—one easy, one hard—use yoga moves. The report includes a special section on additional non-exercise measures you can take to prevent falls.

Cardio Exercise: 7 workouts to boost energy, fight disease, and help you live longer
Lauren E. Elson, M.D., Medical Editor, with Michele Stanten, Fitness Consultant
(Harvard Medical School, 2018)

Looking for cardio workouts? This report will help you find the perfect routine—whether you are just beginning, need to freshen up a routine, or are ready to take your cardio workouts to the next level. There's something for everyone, including kickboxing, step, dance, and interval workouts.

Gentle Core Exercises: Start toning your abs, building your back muscles, and reclaiming core fitness today
Lauren E. Elson, M.D., Medical Editor, with Michele Stanten, Fitness Consultant
(Harvard Medical School, 2017)

When standard core workouts are too challenging—perhaps because you've been ill or you're afraid of aggravating an injury—the workouts in *Gentle Core Exercises* can provide solutions. The report even includes simple exercises and stretches that can be done at the office.

Strength and Power Training for All Ages: 4 complete workouts to tone up, slim down, and get fit
Elizabeth Pegg Frates, M.D., Medical Editor, with Michele Stanten, Fitness Consultant
(Harvard Medical School, 2017)

These four complete workouts allow you to progress from easy to hard strength and power exercises. The report includes a basic workout plus workouts using different types of equipment—resistance bands, a medicine ball, and kettlebell. For bonus work on power training, there is also a section on plyometrics.

Walking for Health: Why this simple form of activity could be your best health insurance
Lauren E. Elson, M.D., Medical Editor, with Michele Stanten, Fitness Consultant
(Harvard Medical School, 2019)

Walking is one of the simplest forms of exercise—and one of the best. This report includes five different walking workouts, information on proper technique, tips on finding the right shoes and socks, safety pointers, and more.